100 Questions & Answers About Sinusitis and Other Sinus Diseases

Rhoda Wynn, MD
California Sinus Institute

Winston C. Vaughan, MD
California Sinus Institute

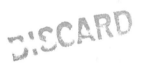

JONES AND BARTLETT PUBLISHERS
Sudbury, Massachusetts
BOSTON   TORONTO   LONDON   SINGAPORE

World Headquarters
Jones and Bartlett Publishers
40 Tall Pine Drive
Sudbury, MA 01776
978-443-5000
info@jbpub.com
www.jbpub.com

Jones and Bartlett Publishers
Canada
6339 Ormindale Way
Mississauga, Ontario
L5V 1J2
CANADA

Jones and Bartlett Publishers
International
Barb House, Barb Mews
London W6 7PA
UK

Jones and Bartlett's books and products are available through most bookstores and online booksellers. To contact Jones and Bartlett Publishers directly, call 800-832-0034, fax 978-443-8000, or visit our website www.jbpub.com.

Substantial discounts on bulk quantities of Jones and Bartlett's publications are available to corporations, professional associations, and other qualified organizations. For details and specific discount information, contact the special sales department at Jones and Bartlett via the above contact information or send an email to specialsales@jbpub.com.

The authors, editor, and publisher have made every effort to provide accurate information. However, they are not responsible for errors, omissions, or for any outcomes related to the use of the contents of this book and take no responsibility for the use of the products described. Treatments and side effects described in this book may not be applicable to all patients; likewise, some patients may require a dose or experience a side effect that is not described herein. The reader should confer with his or her own physician regarding specific treatments and side effects. Drugs and medical devices are discussed that may have limited availability controlled by the Food and Drug Administration (FDA) for use only in a research study or clinical trial. The drug information presented has been derived from reference sources, recently published data, and pharmaceutical research data. Research, clinical practice, and government regulations often change the accepted standard in this field. When consideration is being given to use of any drug in the clinical setting, the health care provider or reader is responsible for determining FDA status of the drug, reading the package insert, reviewing prescribing information for the most up-to-date recommendations on dose, precautions, and contraindications, and determining the appropriate usage for the product. This is especially important in the case of drugs that are new or seldom used.

Library of Congress Cataloging-in-Publication Data

Wynn, Rhoda H.
  100 questions and answers about sinusitis and other sinus diseases / Rhoda Wynn and Winston C. Vaughan.
    p. cm.
  Includes index.
  ISBN-13: 978-0-7637-4305-5
  ISBN-10: 0-7637-4305-4
  1. Sinusitis—Popular works. 2. Paranasal sinuses—Diseases—Popular works. I. Vaughan, Winston C. II. Title.
III. Title: One hundred questions and answers about sinusitis and other sinus diseases.
  RF425.W96 2008
  616.2'12—dc22
                        2007028154
6048

Production Credits

Executive Publisher: Christopher Davis
Associate Editor: Kathy Richardson
Production Director: Amy Rose
Associate Production Editor: Mike Boblitt
Associate Marketing Manager: Rebecca Wasley
Manufacturing Buyer: Therese Connell

Cover Design: Jon Ayotte
Composition: Spoke & Wheel/Jason Miranda
Cover Image: © Photos.com
Printing and Binding: Malloy, Inc.
Cover Printing: Malloy, Inc.

Printed in the United States of America
11 10 09 08 07   10 9 8 7 6 5 4 3 2 1

We dedicate this to you, our patients facing sinusitis, and your families. We hope that this book is both interesting and informative. Thank you for allowing us the privilege of caring for you.

CONTENTS

Sinusitis is one of the most common medical problems from which patients suffer. Most patients are treated successfully in the primary care setting by family practice physicians, internists, pediatricians, or emergency room physicians. Some patients ultimately are evaluated and treated by specialists in allergy/immunology or otorhinolaryngology.

Sinusitis is not a single disorder but several different conditions for which the underlying causes have not been fully delineated. It should therefore not be surprising that patients misunderstand sinusitis and have many questions. Diverse specialists answer patient questions in different ways. Answers vary depending on the specific kind of sinusitis a patient has, and doctors don't fully understand sinusitis themselves. Now, Drs. Wynn and Vaughan, specialists in sinusitis, provide comprehensive answers to 100 common questions patients ask about sinusitis and sinusitis treatment.

This book offers important information for patients in a format that is easy to use. It is divided into eight parts that address key topics such as sinusitis diagnosis, management, sinus surgery, and alternative therapies. Part 3 provides an especially helpful section for patients on what to expect during a visit to the doctor's office for sinusitis. Part 6 offers valuable information about living with sinusitis and gives tips for preventing sinus infections. Thorough, yet easy to understand, answers are provided in a practical format.

This book is the best patient resource available that addresses the most commonly asked patient questions about sinusitis. It is a valuable asset to patients with sinusitis and to health care providers caring for patients with sinus disease. Drs. Wynn and Vaughan are to be congratulated for their excellent contribution to patients through this book.

William E. Bolger, MD
Maryland Sinus Center
Bethesda, Maryland

Sinusitis is a common, and often difficult to treat, problem for many people. We have sought additional training in caring for patients with sinusitis and manage many people with sinusitis in our medical practices. Working on this book has allowed us to share our knowledge and has also given us additional personal insight into these diseases as we delved into its impact on our patients during the writing process. We hope this book will engage and inform our patients and the many others who suffer from sinusitis and related disorders.

In the United States, sinusitis is one of the most common reasons for people to miss work and require the care of a physician. There is a broad spectrum of disease, ranging from short-lived "cold-like" episodes to lifelong disease that must be managed much like high blood pressure or diabetes. For the unfortunate subset of patients with chronic sinusitis, it can be profoundly debilitating, perhaps more so because its presence is not immediately obvious to the casual observer.

Fortunately, the medical profession understands progressively more about how sinusitis develops and what its causes are. There are effective therapies now for sinusitis, though there are no cures at this point. This book is designed to provide you with insight into sinusitis and related disorders and to help guide you in your attempts at achieving control over the disease.

ACKNOWLEDGMENTS

We would like thank Justin Ortiz, MD, for providing illustrations for this book. We would also like to thank the patients who took the time to review our book and for sharing their experiences in the patient commentary sections.

PART ONE

Getting Started: The Basics of Sinusitis

What are the sinuses?

How do the normal nose and sinuses function?

Why do we have sinuses?

More . . .

1: What are the sinuses?

Sinuses

Hollow air-filled cavities located in the head.

A person is usually born with the maxillary and ethmoid sinuses, and the frontal and sphenoid sinuses develop gradually as you grow older, with growth nearly complete during the late teens.

Frontal sinus

Sinus located in the forehead above the eyes.

Dura sinus

Thick, tough covering that surrounds and protects the brain.

Ethmoid sinus

Sinus composed of many small cells located between the eyes.

Maxillary sinus

Sinus located in the cheeks on either side of the nose.

The **sinuses** are hollow cavities in the head. There can be up to eight air-containing cavities inside your skull up to four pairs of sinuses present. These are the frontal, ethmoid, maxillary, and sphenoid sinuses. One of each sinus is located on the right and one on the left of your face, and they surround the eyes. A person is usually born with the maxillary and ethmoid sinuses, and the frontal and sphenoid sinuses develop gradually as you grow older, with growth nearly complete during the late teens. The fully developed sinuses often vary in size, and sometimes shape, from one side to the other. Some sinuses may fail to develop, but the absence of these sinuses does not usually create a problem.

The sinuses in the forehead, located directly above the eyes, are called the **frontal** sinuses. They are located directly in front of the brain and are separated from the brain by the back bony wall of the sinus and a thick covering that surrounds the brain called the **dura**.

The sinuses located between the eyes and behind the bridge of the nose are called the ethmoid sinuses. The **ethmoid** sinuses are comprised of many small air-containing spaces interconnected like a honeycomb. They are in the space under the brain from the front to the back of the nasal cavity. These sinuses have the thinnest bones making up their structure. Also, their outer walls serve as the thin barriers that separate them from surrounding structures such as the eye and the brain.

The pair of sinuses located underneath the eyes and on either side of the nostrils are called the **maxillary** sinuses. These are the sinuses in closest proximity to the teeth. They are also the ones that most often cause sinus discomfort.

The set of sinuses deepest inside the head, furthest behind the eyes and also under the brain, are called the **sphenoid** sinuses. They are essentially in the center of the head. They may lie very close in association to the optic nerve, which controls vision, and internal carotid arteries, which supply blood to the brain. Often, the bones between these structures and the sinuses can be very thin or these structures may run through the sinus air spaces.

Sphenoid sinus
Sinus located deep inside the head, under the brain and behind the eyes.

The frontal, maxillary, and ethmoid sinuses that line up in the frontal plane drain through a set of channels that are in the anterior aspect of the nose. The sphenoids and some of the deeper ethmoids drain further back in the nose. The locations of the sinuses are shown in front and side plane cross sections in **Figures 1** and **2**.

2. How do the normal nose and sinuses function?

The nose is the air conditioner for the lungs. After we inhale air, it is warmed during the passage through the nasal cavity into the windpipe and lungs. The air is also humidified and filtered during this time. Structures called **turbinates**, which are long shelf-like structures made of bone and mucosa, help increase the surface area available for the exchange of heat and moisture for warming and humidification during the movement of air through the nose. In most people, there are three sets of turbinates: superior, middle, and inferior. A small number of people may have a fourth set, called the supreme turbinates. The turbinates are oriented horizontally in the nasal cavity, parallel with the floor of the nose or the roof of the mouth. **Figure 3** shows the sinuses and turbinates in cross section from the side, and **Figure 4** shows them in cross section from the front.

The nose is the air conditioner for the lungs.

Turbinates
Scrolls of bone covered with mucosa that extend from the nasal walls inside the nose that humidify and warm the air as it passes through the nasal passageway.

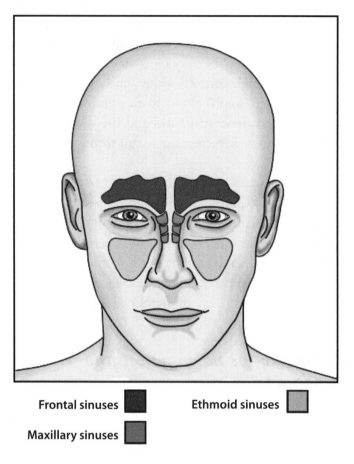

Frontal sinuses ■   Ethmoid sinuses ■

Maxillary sinuses ■

Figure 1 Location of the sinuses: frontal view

Mucosal membrane

Thin layer of tissue that lines normal nose and sinuses.

Cilia

Microscopic hairs on the surface of the mucosa lining of the nose and sinuses that beat in a synchronized fashion to help sweep away mucus and debris.

Mucus

Fluid secreted from the cells lining the nose and sinuses.

The normal nose and sinuses are lined with a thin layer of tissue called the **mucosal membrane**. This is like the lining inside your cheeks that at times may lift off after a burn. The outer layer of this sinus and nasal mucosal membrane is covered with tiny hairs, which are called **cilia**. These hairs will move like the legs of a centipede in a coordinated fashion. These cilia beat in a single direction toward the drainage pathway of that particular sinus. A thin layer of **mucus**, produced by the sinuses, sits on top of the cilia and is swept by the motion of the cilia out toward the opening of the sinus. The mucus

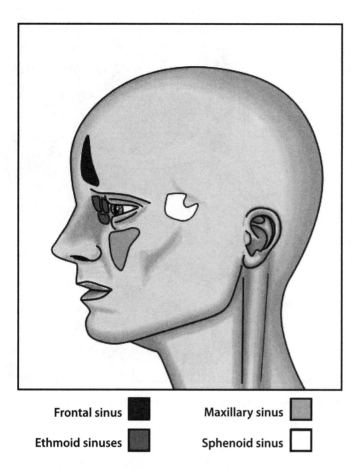

| Frontal sinus | ■ | Maxillary sinus | ■ |
| Ethmoid sinuses | ■ | Sphenoid sinus | □ |

Figure 2 Location of the sinuses: side view

normally is thin and is needed for normal sinus and lung function. It serves several roles including the humidification and warming of the air that we breathe through our noses. Imagine what would happen if our delicate lungs were not exposed to warm and moist air on a regular basis.

The sinus openings through which the sinus secretions drain into the nasal cavities are called **ostia**. They are like very small doorways to large rooms. The ostia of the maxillary sinuses under the eyes are actually located in

Ostia

Small openings from the sinuses into the nasal cavities.

5

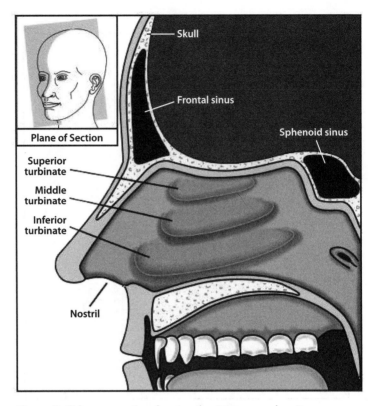

Figure 3 Side cross section showing the sinuses, nasal cavity, and the turbinates

the upper parts of their walls, while the other sinuses may have their doorways located in their floors or a lower side wall. Ostia are often only 1–2 millimeters in size and often represent the weak point for sinuses. When things go wrong at the ostia, the rest of the sinus may malfunction.

Mucociliary clearance

The process by which mucus and materials caught within it are moved from the nose and sinuses by the cilia to the back of the throat.

The mucus in the sinuses eventually drains in small and continuous quantities down the back of the nose and into the throat, after which it is swallowed and passed into the stomach. The process of sinus self-cleaning is called **mucociliary clearance**. It's similar to the windshield cleaning system of a car with the wipers serving as

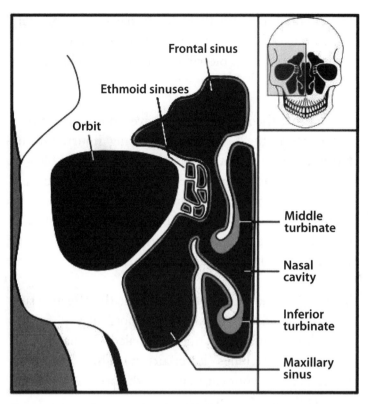

Figure 4 Frontal cross section showing the sinuses and the turbinates

the cilia and the washer fluid as the mucus. Dust, pollen, bacteria, and other inhaled particles get trapped in the mucus and are cleared out by this process.

3: Why do we have sinuses?

Doctors are not sure what the exact reasons are for the head to contain these air-containing spaces. However, there are several possibilities or theories. One theory is that the hollow spaces of the sinuses may help the voice resonate and affect the sound of speech. Another theory is that they may help to lighten the weight of the skull, allowing humans to evolve in some advantageous way.

Other possibilities are that sinuses may serve as pressure release valves for the dramatic changes in pressure experienced during nose blowing, sneezing, or rapid changes in altitude.

Yet another theory for why we have sinuses is that they can serve as the brain's airbag during injury. During facial trauma, the sinuses absorb the impact of a blow to the head and act as "crumple zones" that decrease deeper injury to the more important structures of the eyes and brain. This theory is believed by many to be the most clinically relevant one, along with the sinus's role in air filtering, which will be explained later.

The sinuses may also serve to increase the effective surface area inside the nasal cavity (upper airway) for the humidification and heating of inhaled air that is then carried into the lungs (lower airway). This is similar to the radiator of your car that does the opposite by cooling the fluid in the engine.

Other suggestions that have been proposed are that sinus tissue serves as a framework over which some nerve fibers for smell and associations with taste lie. These cells and nerve endings, are the key component of the olfactory (smell) system's interaction with the outside world. The sinus tissue and its mucus may serve to increase the surface area for exposure to outside element particles with the nerves and hence enhance the ability to smell.

Mucus is a useful fluid secreted from the cells and glands lining the nose and sinuses.

4: What is mucus made of and what does it do?

As just mentioned, sinus mucus is normal. It is a fluid we all produce. Mucus is a useful fluid secreted from the cells and glands lining the nose and sinuses. It traps the particles that are floating through the nose into a solution when we inhale. These particles are then transported into the throat within the mucus, and fewer of these particles pass into the lungs. This filtration role is also a crucial function of the mucus produced by the sinuses. It helps with foreign particle clearance from the airway—like the air filter for your car; when it malfunctions, the lungs (engine) may also have problems.

Sinus and nasal mucus is composed of water, proteins, salts, and enzymes. Many of these enzymes and proteins are protective and help with the body's continuous interaction with the outside world. These enzymes react to and defend against allergens, viruses, bacteria, fungal organisms, and countless chemicals and particles.

The nose makes about 2 liters of mucus daily. Yes, you read that correctly; a large soda bottle amount of mucus per day is pumped out of your nose and sinuses into the upper airway. This mucus is propelled at a rate of 3 to 25 mm per minute toward the sinus ostia and down into the lower airway and throat.

Sinusitis occurs when the lining of the sinuses, called the mucosa, becomes inflamed or irritated.

5: What is sinusitis?

Sinusitis is a large group of diseases of the sinus lining and sometimes the surrounding structures. Sinusitis occurs when the lining of the sinuses, called the mucosa, becomes inflamed or irritated. The inflammation of the lining of the sinuses can become so extensive that it causes the very small sinus ostia to become blocked. Normal mucociliary clearance, previously discussed, cannot occur. The obstructed ostia trap the mucus within the sinuses. The arrows in **Figure 5** show normal mucociliary clearance on the right side and show mucus accumulation from blocked flow on the left side.

Sinusitis

Disease characterized by inflammation of the mucosa lining the sinuses.

9

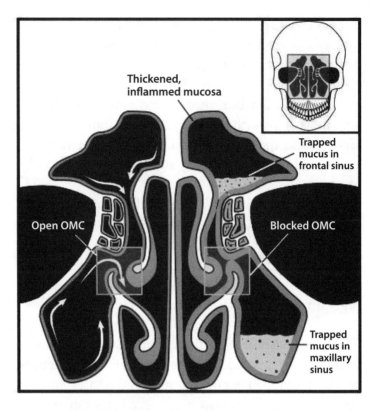

Figure 5 Normal mucociliary clearance is shown by the arrows on the right-sided sinuses. The left side shows mucus trapped by blocked sinus drainage pathways.

Sinuses are warm, dark spaces that when filled with wet mucus can create the conditions that are perfect for organisms to grow. These are the conditions that are also ideal for fungal organisms to grow. There are other warm, dark, and moist spaces that fungus grows well in; for example, under wet carpet, in the bathroom, and under the refrigerator.

Bacteria

A type of micro-organism that can cause infection.

The infectious **bacterial** and fungal organisms can themselves cause additional tissue irritation and swelling or inflammation that slows normal mucus clearance within the sinus, further propagating the cycle of inflammation and infection. Sinus cavities that are infected and/or swollen cause the major symptoms that most people call sinusitis.

6: What are the causes of sinusitis?

Anatomic, genetic, and environmental factors can all contribute individually, but often jointly, to the development of sinusitis. Anatomic factors are those that affect the shapes of the sinus drainage pathways. Genetic factors include how your body's enzymes and proteins react. Environmental factors are the outside factors that can influence the sinuses.

An overgrowth of normal organisms or new growth of unusual organisms can lead to an infection in the sinus cavities. The infection in sinusitis may be caused by either fungal or bacterial organisms, or even both types present at the same time. Sinusitis often develops after a cold, when the lining of the nose and sinuses becomes inflamed. This leads to swelling of the drainage pathways, and the sinus ostia becomes blocked.

Aside from blocked sinus ostia, anatomic causes include variations in the structure of the nose and sinuses that may also predispose to sinusitis. Drainage of the frontal, maxillary, and sphenoid sinuses may be blocked by the various types of ethmoid sinus cells that grow into narrow spaces and tighten or limit the openings even more. For instance, an ethmoid sinus cell called a Haller cell can grow into the part of the maxillary sinus closest to the inside of the nasal cavity and narrow the drainage pathway of the maxillary sinus.

The major sinuses in the front of the nose, which are the ethmoid, maxillary, and frontal sinuses, all drain into a similar pathway. This area is called the ostiomeatal complex region. This region can also be narrowed by a deviated nasal septum or enlargement of the turbinates, discussed in the **Questions 26** and **27**.

Hereditary disorders such as cystic fibrosis (CF) may cause patients to be prone to develop sinusitis. Other factors may predispose patients to sinus problems. Certain autoimmune diseases may also have nasal manifestations and predispose patients to sinusitis. Immunocompromised states caused either by medications such as long-term steroid therapy or chemotherapy, human immunodeficiency virus (HIV) infection, or chronic illnesses such as diabetes may also predispose patients to sinus infections.

Environmental factors that can contribute to sinusitis include exposure to smoke. Dust in the home can be a problem for people with dust-mite allergies. Irritants such as pollution can increase inflammation within the nasal cavity.

Sinusitis, which is an upper respiratory tract infection, can be contagious, because the organisms causing sinusitis can become airborne.

7: Can I give sinusitis to other people?

Sinusitis, which is an upper respiratory tract infection, can be contagious, because the organisms causing sinusitis can become airborne. It is like a cold where the nasal fluid can be passed to surfaces that others may touch as may occur after a sneeze. It is for this reason that you should always cover your mouth and nose when sneezing and coughing. The bacteria can also be spread through other contacts like facial tissues. The best practice to decrease transmission of microbes is frequent handwashing. Antimicrobial soaps and gels are also extremely useful in decreasing the spread of infections. Experts strongly recommend that hand washing be performed consistently when ill. Often, however, by the time you actually experience symptoms of an infection, the organisms have been shared with others. Fortunately, most people can fight off a mild exposure. This does not apply to very young children, patients with immune disorders, or those receiving chemotherapy who are immunosuppressed. Avoid contact with such persons if you are very sick with an acute sinus infection because they are more vulnerable to infectious disease.

Chronic sinusitis is less likely to be contagious because it is often due to inflammation and swelling. However, chronic sinus patients can also develop recurring infections. These infections can also include unusual or drug-resistant strains of organisms. Therefore, all patients need to be vigilant about hygiene. When patients are sick and the infection does not seem to respond to treatment, most doctors recommend a sinus culture to help determine what the organisms are and what drugs may be used to kill it. See **Question 35**.

8: Is sinusitis common?

Most of us have had one or more sinus infections at some point. This often occurs following a cold: when the cold just does not seem to go away and other localized symptoms, such as increased facial pain or tenderness over the sinuses, start to occur in the face. According to statistics from the National Center for Health Statistics, approximately 29–35 million American adults annually in the years from 1995–2005, suffered from chronic sinusitis. Most of these infections are brief and acute—often less than 10 days—infections that often may resolve by themselves. However, these can persist, making sinus infections one of the most common diagnoses for which antibiotics are prescribed and frequent reasons for patients to visit a doctor or urgent care provider.

In 2002, according to the Sinus and Allergy Health Partnership, sinusitis accounted for about 9 percent of pediatric and 21 percent of adult antibiotic prescriptions. Tracking the use of antibiotics for sinus infections and other upper respiratory tract infections serves as a vital source of information on the rates of infections that the population experiences. It also sheds light concerning the emergence of antibiotic resistant bacteria in the general population.

Because of the large numbers of people who may be affected by sinus infections, chronic sinusitis also has significant impact on work productivity. Many of us know what happens when several people in an office come down with upper respiratory infections at the same time. There are also very convincing reports obtained through patient surveys that show that impact on quality of life is worse in perceived body pain and social functioning than chronic obstructive pulmonary disease, congestive heart failure, angina (chest pain), and back pain.

9: What is the difference between acute, subacute, and chronic sinusitis?

Sinusitis is often classified into three groups that are determined by the duration of the illness.

Acute sinusitis infections most often last less than 6 weeks. This is the most common type of sinus infection. Many of us have already experienced what these may feel

Acute sinusitis
Sinus infections that last less than 6 weeks.

like, including the drainage, facial pain, and pressure that often come with these infections. This is most common after a cold (virus) that gets more complex when a bacterial infection gets involved also. A course of antibiotic medications may be needed to treat these infections.

Subacute sinus infections last between 6 to 12 weeks. These are considered to be persistent acute infections that often have a fair amount of swelling (inflammation) as a result of the tissue response to the first acute infection. Fatigue, cough, a decreased sense of smell, and nasal blockage are the symptoms that are most common in the subacute patient.

Chronic sinusitis infections are those that last longer than 12 weeks. Patients with chronic infections present to ear, nose, and throat (ENT) surgeons because the infections have failed to clear up after many courses of different medications. These patients are often considering surgery for sinus drainage. The "infections" may actually no longer be due to bacterial infection. They are more likely due to the tissues' being chronically swollen or inflamed, which then closes the sinus drainage holes (ostia) and does not allow clearance of the normal sinus fluids. These fluids may then get secondarily infected. This cycle of infection leading to inflammation and then inflammation leading to more infection is the vicious circle that envelops chronic patients. For many chronic patients, this circle has to be broken at more than one point to make them better.

Chronic sinusitis
Persistent sinus infection and inflammation lasting 12 weeks or more.

10: Can sinusitis be cured?

Acute sinusitis is treated with a course of antibiotic pills. Most of the milder episodes of acute sinus infection can actually resolve on their own without prescribed medicines. The body's immune system kicks in to fight off these infections. Patients will also self-treat with over-the-counter medications to decrease some of the symptoms while the body deals with the infection. Most acute episodes are cured by the body itself or with the help of a course of medications.

Subacute infections are more difficult to cure and treat. They often require several weeks of treatment. They may also require courses of steroids to help decrease the swelling of the tissues to open the ostia and drainage pathways.

Chronic sinusitis is the most difficult to treat. It is not curable, but treatment can decrease many of the symptoms to tolerable levels. Patients with chronic sinusitis will often present with a wide range of symptoms, some of which are treatable. However, some symptoms may be due to the sinus tissues being damaged. As an example, some patients with chronic sinusitis will lose their sense of smell, and sometimes taste, due to damage to the nerves at the top of the nose during the illness.

Chronic sinusitis is very similar to diabetes and hypertension in the sense that ongoing treatment is needed to control the symptoms of the disease.

At this time, there is no definitive cure for chronic sinusitis. Chronic sinusitis is very similar to diabetes and hypertension in the sense that ongoing treatment is needed to control the symptoms of the disease. Good control of disease can be achieved through a combination of medical and surgical therapy. A commitment must be made to disease management by the patient, because maintenance therapy is required to prevent relapse of the disease and keep the sinuses as calm as possible.

11: What are nasal polyps?

Nasal polyps are pink, watery-appearing growths that occur within the nose and sinuses. They look like blisters of the tissue and when removed may look like small grapes. **Figure 6** shows some nasal polyps inside a nasal cavity. Polyps are sometimes seen in conjunction with allergies or sinusitis. They range in size from very small swellings that do not cause much trouble and sit on the outer aspects of the sinuses while other polyps may grow in key drainage points and though small can lead to critical blockage. Larger polyps can completely fill the nasal cavity and be visible from looking through the nostrils.

Sinus and nasal polyps are not like polyps in other parts of the body, such as the colon (large intestine). They are almost always benign and not a precursor to cancer. However, there are growths in the sinuses and nose that may look like polyps but can be precancerous growths or, in rare cases, contain cancer. Precancerous and cancerous

Nasal polyps
Pink, watery growths that can develop in the nose and sinuses.

Nasal polyps are pink, watery-appearing growths that occur within the nose and sinuses.

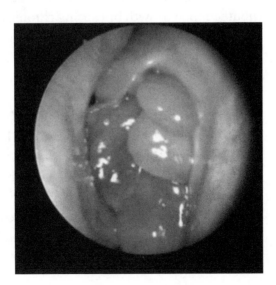

Figure 6
Nasal polyps

17

masses usually grow only on one side of the nose, while most true benign nasal polyps are present in both sides. Polyps present in one nasal cavity, but not the other, should be biopsied or removed, especially if there are other factors that make them more suspicious.

Inverted papilloma

Noncancerous, but aggressively growing tumor of the nose and sinuses.

For instance, there is a type of wart-like growth that looks similar to a polyp and is called an **inverted papilloma**. These are most often benign. However, they do not shrink in response to steroids as benign nasal polyps do. According to several otolaryngology textbooks, about 10–15 percent of inverted papillomas may be associated with sinus cancer.

12: What causes nasal polyps?

The exact cause of benign nasal polyps is unknown at this time, but there are multiple factors that may contribute to their growth. These polyps may represent the final result of chronic inflammation. Allergies may contribute to their growth by causing chronic inflammation of the tissues. Patients with fungal sinus infections often have severe allergic reactions to the fungus, and their sinuses may have the most extensive polyps.

Asthma

A disorder in which the lungs become inflamed and constrict in response to triggers such as dust, pollens, pollution, cold temperatures or exercise.

Patients with **asthma** (which causes problems with the linings of the breathing passageways) are known to have a higher probability of having nasal polyps. A hereditary component or cause for polyps may also be suspected in some patients. As an example, some CF patients have nasal polyps. In general, nasal polyps seem to occur more frequently in those with affected family members.

13: What is fungal sinusitis?

Fungal sinusitis represents infection with the fungus, commonly called **mold**, in the paranasal sinuses. The sinuses—like under a carpet in the basement—are warm, dark, and damp. This is the perfect environment for mold to grow.

The least invasive form of fungal sinusitis is called a **fungus ball**. This occurs when a small amount of fungus gets trapped within a sinus. When it grows within the dark and moist space, it can fill the space and obstruct the drainage from the sinus without invading the tissue. The expanding fungus may even push on the bone and cause it to be thinned or expand in size or become distorted in shape. This type of fungal infection typically involves only one sinus. Medications are insufficient for the treatment of a fungus ball. Medications have no effect on fungus balls because they are not attached to or invading the tissue and into the blood supply of the sinus cavity, so antibiotics in the bloodstream cannot penetrate it. The sinus must be surgically opened and the fungus ball removed, often by just lifting it out or flushing the sinus clear.

There is a much more serious type of fungal sinus infection, but it is rare. This form of fungal sinusitis is called **invasive fungal sinusitis**. It occurs most frequently in patients with poor immune systems like diabetics or patients undergoing chemotherapy. This type of fungal infection is often caused by a fungus called either *mucor* or *aspergillus*. The infection that develops invades the bone and soft tissues of the sinuses. The infection is extremely

Fungal sinusitis represents infection with the fungus, commonly called mold, in the paranasal sinuses.

Mold

Fungus; plants that make spores instead of seeds.

Fungus ball

Form of fungal sinusitis also called a *mycetoma*, which is a collection of fungal debris within a sinus.

Invasive fungal sinusitis

Aggressive form of fungal sinusitis that develops in immuno-compromised patients and diabetic patients; it rapidly destroys tissue and can spread to the brain and the eye.

destructive and rapid because it destroys nerves and blood vessels as it invades the tissue. The infection can spread to the surrounding structures of the brain and the eyes quickly and is therefore a life-threatening infection. Invasive fungal sinusitis is treated with urgent, extensive, and aggressive surgical removal of all diseased tissue. A surrounding layer of normal tissue may need to be removed to ensure that the invading disease is completely removed.

Allergic fungal sinusitis

Form of sinusitis that is characterized by an allergy to fungus, nasal polyps, and the presence of allergic mucin, a thick peanut butter-like mucus.

The most common and least understood type of sinusitis involving fungus is called **allergic fungal sinusitis (AFS)** and is discussed here.

14: What is allergic fungal sinusitis (AFS)?

Allergic fungal sinusitis is the least understood form of fungal sinusitis. The specific characteristics, findings, means of diagnosis, and treatment options are furiously debated by allergists and ENT doctors. The most commonly agreed-upon criteria include nasal polyps, the presence of thick allergic mucus (called **mucin**), specific X-ray findings, and a documented allergy to fungus. Allergic mucin is sometimes described as a thick, "peanut-butter–like" or "spongy" mucus. This has a characteristic microscopic appearance and can completely fill the sinuses in patients with allergic fungal sinusitis. Fortunately, it is not as serious as invasive fungal sinusitis, but it may also cause bony changes and expansion of the sinus wall into other tissues.

Mucin

Thick, greenish material produced in the sinuses in allergic fungal sinusitis.

Allergic fungal sinusitis can be difficult to diagnose. The diagnosis is often made only after failure of multiple treatments including antibiotics or sinus surgery. It may even be missed by cultures of the mucus because many labs do not search for the fungus or the way the culture was obtained was inadequate.

Once a diagnosis of AFS is made, steroid pills are given to try to decrease the swelling and allow the mucus to drain out of the sinuses. Often, this alone may not solve the problem and patients will be taken to surgery. Surgery is done to remove the obstructing and inflamed mucosal tissue and to allow the removal of the fungus from the sinus. After such initial treatments, AFS patients are often in need of multiple treatments to prevent the disease from recurring. These may include steroid pills, sprays or washes, allergy therapy against certain molds, removal of as much mold from their environment as possible, and close endoscopic monitoring of the sinus cavities. Some patients may also need courses of antifungal pills, washes, or sprays. Secondary bacterial infections and polyp growth are often associated with recurrences in AFS patients.

PART TWO

Diagnosing Sinusitis: Symptoms, Risk Factors, and Related Disorders

What are the symptoms of sinusitis?

How do I tell the difference between
a cold and sinusitis?

Is the color of the mucus from my nose significant?

More . . .

15: What are the symptoms of sinusitis?

Major symptoms of a sinus infection include facial pain or pressure. Sinus pain and pressure are caused by pressure on the nerves of the sinuses by the swollen and irritated tissues. If a polyp or fungus is involved, there is often less pressure and pain compared with acute bacterial infections. Negative pressure vacuum of the sinuses can be caused by blockage of the sinus ostia, and this can result in the symptoms of pain and pressure.

Other major symptoms that may be noted include nasal stuffiness or fullness and pus draining from the front of the nose or down the throat. Many will notice difficulty with the ability to smell and even detect changes in their sense of taste. Swollen nasal tissues and increased or thickened nasal sections can cause difficulty breathing through the nose. Some patients will snore due to this blockage. Other factors evaluated in the diagnosis of sinusitis include headache and bad breath, fatigue, cough, dental pain, and in the case of acute infections, fever. The bad breath is due to the presence of bacteria in the thick mucus that may drain into the throat from the back of the nose during sinusitis.

Tina's comments:

When I have a bout of sinusitis, I usually feel miserable and tired. Often, I have painful headaches above my right eye. My cheeks are very sensitive to touch. I can't smell or taste. My nose is very stuffy, and I can't breathe through it. Blowing my nose brings no relief because all the mucus seems stuck in my head. My ears are achy and can "pop"— and hurt— when I blow my nose. Sleeping is very difficult because of the discomfort and headaches. Raising my head with pillows, almost a sitting position, helps. If I lower my head, the pounding increases.

Paula's comments:

I've had sinus problems all my life. I was tired and frustrated. I had headaches, mostly in the morning, and a stuffy nose. My teeth hurt and my ears plugged up. I had no taste or smell and always slept in an upright position. Nothing seemed to help me feel better.

16: How do I tell the difference between a cold and sinusitis?

It can be difficult to distinguish between having a cold and having sinusitis. Colds are caused by common viruses. Your body's natural defenses usually can fight off these in about a week. However, sinusitis typically has a more protracted course, and the symptoms will persist beyond 5 to 7 days. In fact, sinusitis often will follow or complicate a cold; it's like a cold that doesn't go away. There may be differences in the appearance of the mucus draining from the nose. Many of the over-the-counter treatments available for a cold will help lessen some of the symptoms of a sinus infection, but if bacteria or fungus are present in "infection-level" quantities, symptoms will continue and medical attention is needed.

It can be difficult to distinguish between having a cold and having sinusitis.

Tina's comments:

Because I am very susceptible to sinusitis, if I get a cold, it is almost guaranteed that I get sinusitis. After 2 weeks of a totally stuffed nose and feeling miserable, I know that I have an infection.

Paula's comments:

I never get colds. If I feel cold-like symptoms, it's always a sinus infection.

17: Is the color of the mucus from my nose significant?

Sometimes the color of the mucus from the nose can help with the diagnosis. Viral infection frequently has clear drainage. Allergic rhinitis or "allergies" also usually result in clear drainage. A thick white drainage is often pus, and thick yellow or green drainage may represent a bacterial infection. The draining fluid is thickened by the presence of bacteria and white blood cells fighting the infection in the mucus. However, due to shedding of white blood cells and skin within the mucus, it is possible to have yellow or green drainage during a viral infection. Often, when the infection has been treated and gone, the mucus may stay discolored for a few days or even weeks as the sinuses continue to clear out the old mucus. Some doctors prefer to culture the mucus in the lab and use those data to determine whether there is clinically significant infection versus a colonization of the tissue with normal bacterial flora.

18: What is a sinus headache?

Each of the sinuses has a different nerve supply for pain. The affected sinus often can be identified from the distribution of pain on the face and head that a patient describes. Facial pain and pressure caused by infection of the sinuses will manifest itself as pain above the eyes in patients with frontal sinusitis. Pain and pressure between the eyes is observed in patients with ethmoid sinusitis. Pain and pressure in the cheeks or teeth may be felt in patients with maxillary sinusitis. Diffuse or generalized pain in the back of the head or pain behind the eyes may be seen in patients with sphenoid sinusitis.

Tina's comments:

My sinus headaches were originally diagnosed as stress and tension headaches. It was finally recognized that I was actually suffering from sinus headaches only after treatment for the other types of headaches did not work. When having an acute attack, I feel like there is extreme pressure that can be pinpointed to an area in my head, usually above my right eye that causes terrible pain. I sometimes wish I could drill into my head at that spot to relieve the pressure. Aspirin or other nonsteroidal anti-inflammatory agents (NSAIDs) like ibuprofen are not effective in treating the pain.

Paula's comments:

I've had migraines all my life. Before my sinus surgeries, I had two or three migraines per month. Now I have maybe two or three a year. I still have a lot of sinus headaches. I usually wake up with them, and they are always above my eyes.

19: What are other causes of sinus headaches and facial pain?

Headaches and facial pain are nonspecific symptoms; many different diseases can cause one to feel a headache and have facial pain, not just sinusitis. Headaches can pinpoint a problem to the head, but often there is not much further beyond that in identifying specific cause that you can say from the symptom. Seek medical assistance for frequent, persistent, or unexplained headaches.

Migraine headaches and cluster headaches may be particularly difficult to distinguish from pain caused by sinus diseases. This is because they have symptoms

. . . many different diseases can cause one to feel a headache and have facial pain . . .

Migraine

Severe form of headaches, often one sided that can be mistaken for a sinus headache; can be associated with light sensitivity, nausea, or postnasal drip.

that may overlap with sinus infection, such as nasal congestion or nasal drainage. Migraines in particular are often misdiagnosed as sinusitis and sinus pain. Surprisingly, migraines are present in more than 10 percent of the population; data published from a study from the National Institutes of Health indicated that the prevalence of migraines in the United States was about 121 per 1,000 people during 2006. Vision changes, nausea, and light sensitivity are other symptoms that may suggest migraine headaches. These are rarely seen in patients who have only sinusitis. A variant of migraine headaches, facial migraines, can even cause pain in the cheeks and the forehead. In addition, some types of headaches can cause watery eyes and runny nose to suggest allergy and sinus problems, but they are only a new relay from the brain to the sinus tissues and not the sinuses serving as the source point for this problem. Your sinus doctor may send you to a neurology (nerve) doctor to help distinguish the type of headache syndromes that may be involved, and likewise neurologists often send their patients to sinus doctors to make sure that the sinuses are not a contributing factor.

Examples of nervous system disorders that can mimic sinusitis include:

1. *Neuritis:* an inflammation of nerve endings that triggers pain; viral infections and trauma are some possible causes; it can occur after sinus surgery.

2. *Neuralgias:* intense burning or stabbing pain caused by irritation or damage to a nerve, such as trigeminal neuralgia, which is facial pain in the distribution of a branch of the nerve supplying sensation to the face.

20: What are other causes of a runny nose?

Other causes of a runny nose besides sinusitis may include allergic rhinitis, vasomotor rhinitis, and a viral infection such as a cold. Vasomotor rhinitis occurs when a runny nose is triggered by things such as heat, cold, or spicy foods.

Gastroesophageal reflux (GERD) can cause the sensation of a postnasal drip; GERD occurs when acids and other enzymes from the stomach and esophagus (food pipe) back up into the throat, pool inside the throat, and cause an inflammatory (and sometimes destructive) response. These pooled secretions cause the feeling of mucus or phlegm dripping in the back of the throat, hoarseness, and cough. It seems that the nose and sinuses may respond to GERD by producing more sinus mucus in an attempt to wash down the gastric digestive fluids. Often we need to address both the nose and the esophagus in patients with severe postnasal drip to make a difference.

Paula's comments:

I had surgery for GERD in 2006. I never related my sinus infections to acid reflux, although I'm sure it's probably all related somehow.

21: Why is my sense of smell affected when I have sinusitis?

The nerve tissue that helps with the ability to smell is located in the roof of the nasal cavity on both sides. In addition, it is located along the upper portions of middle and superior turbinates. The turbinates are shelves of tissue along the sides of the nose that act as the humidifiers of the nose. As air is conducted into the nose, it passes over the olfactory epithelium (smell sensors) in the roof of the nasal cavity, which detects smell after it is transferred from particles into solution. These nerve receptors then send signals from the olfactory nerves toward the brain. When your sinuses get inflamed from a cold or some type of infection, the nerves are "buried" under the swollen tissue and cannot pick up the smell particles to send their information to the brain.

22: What makes me susceptible for getting sinusitis?

Any condition that leads to swelling of the lining of the nose or sinuses (inflammation) may make you susceptible for getting sinusitis. These conditions may include allergic rhinitis, chronic rhinitis, inflammatory diseases of the airway such as asthma, diseases of the airway such as CF, immunocompromised state such as HIV infection, chemotherapy, diabetes, or prolonged steroid use. Other structural problems that lead to narrowed pathways also may lead to an increased risk of sinus problems. These may include polyps, enlarged turbinates, deviated septum, or other tissue that leads to blockage of the sinus drainage holes.

23: What is allergic rhinitis?

Allergic rhinitis is a "hyperreactive response" of your nose to normal environmental exposures. These may include inhalants from mold, dust mites, trees, pets, weeds, and grasses. The body makes chemicals in response to these environmental particles. These allergic chemicals are those that are responsible for inflammation and fighting off infections. The release of these

Allergic rhinitis

An inflammation of the lining of the nose triggered by a substance to which sensitivity has been acquired.

Allergic rhinitis is a "hyperreactive response" of your nose to normal environmental exposures.

chemicals can result in nasal congestion, watery eyes, nasal obstruction, runny nose, postnasal drip, and cough. Allergies may be seasonal or perennial (year round). The allergy-induced chemicals released can cause responses in other areas of the body at the same time, including the eyes and lungs.

24: What is nonallergic rhinitis?

Nonallergic rhinitis is a condition in which inflammation in the nasal passageways is caused by chemicals or other adulterants in the environment that are not true allergens. They cannot be tested for under present circumstances. Many of these nonallergens are chemical agents such as perfumes, cigarette smoke, and other air pollutants. It is also possible that common allergens can cause allergy-like symptoms by acting as irritants leading to inflammation rather than provoking the classical allergy response of the body.

Nonallergic rhinitis

Nasal congestion, sneezing, and runny nose triggered by non-allergens such as chemical irritants, hormones, infections, or drugs.

The most common subtype of nonallergic rhinitis is called **vasomotor rhinitis**. This is a condition in which the body responds to certain stimuli such as heat or cold by producing additional mucus from the nose and causing nasal congestion. Many patients with this form of rhinitis may notice that their noses will respond to temperature and barometric pressure changes. One sufferer said: "I feel like a weather girl; my nose can tell when a storm is coming in."

Vasomotor rhinitis

Abnormal response to stimuli such as heat, cold, or spicy foods that results in nasal congestion and rhinorrhea.

Another type of rhinitis can be seen when we have hormonal changes. Hormonal causes of rhinorrhea may include low thyroid hormone or elevated levels of estrogen during pregnancy, the use of oral contraceptives, and the menstrual cycle. Twenty percent of pregnancies have pregnancy-induced rhinitis, usually with onset during the second trimester.

Paula's comments:

I've been tested for allergies several times. My tests are negative. I do react to certain pollens and windy days. Animals don't bother me.

25: How are "allergies" related to sinusitis?

In several published studies, about 80 percent of patients with chronic sinusitis also have allergic rhinitis. Allergies may often precede or trigger episodes of sinusitis. Swelling inside the nose due to inflammation from allergy or an irritant can narrow the small drainage openings of the sinuses, causing them to become blocked. When the sinuses are blocked, the mucus that they normally produce will build up and serve as a medium in which an infection may develop.

Tina's comments:

I have had severe allergies all my life and because of always having a runny, stuffy nose and discolored mucus, I never knew that I had chronic sinusitis.

26: What is a deviated nasal septum?

Nasal septum

Wall made of bone and cartilage that separates the two sides of the nose.

The **nasal septum** is the wall separating the two sides of the nose. This partition is composed of both cartilage and bone and is covered by a thin layer of tissue that has blood vessels running through it. A deviated nasal septum is one that is bent so that it protrudes more into one side of the nose than the other. An example of a deviated nasal septum is shown in **Figure 7**. This can happen for several reasons. In some people, the septum is bent when passing through the birth canal. In others, it gets damaged

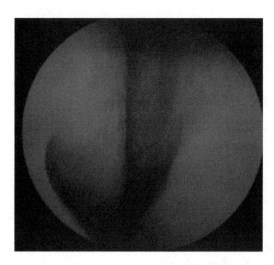

Figure 7
Deviated nasal
septum

when the nose is hit or broken by an injury. A deviated nasal septum can block airflow on the side into which it protrudes. This may lead to a sense of nasal blockage and may even cause snoring.

Another problem with a deviated septum is nosebleeds. When air passes over the area of the deviated septum that is more protruded, it can dry the overlying layer. This layer may then crack and expose the underlying vessels that then bleed. These nosebleeds are quite common and can be stopped by simply applying pressure to the front of the septum by squeezing the nostrils together.

27: What are nasal turbinates, and how do enlarged nasal turbinates cause problems?

The turbinates are sausage-shaped structures made of thin bone covered by spongy mucous membranes in the nasal cavities. There are three on each side called the superior, middle, and inferior turbinates; the turbinates have three main functions. They warm the air we breathe, humidify this air as it passes through the nose, and the mucous layer of the turbinates assists in filtering particles such as dust and pollen.

The turbinates, particularly the inferior, can block breathing when they are enlarged. The inferior turbinates are most commonly enlarged by swelling of the mucous membranes caused by allergies. This enlargement is due to increased blood flow into the tissue that then is "congested." The middle turbinates can be enlarged if an "air bubble" develops inside the bone, a condition called **concha bullosa**. Concha bullosa of the middle turbinates narrows the space through which the sinuses drain, the ostiomeatal complex, and hence can contribute to sinusitis.

Concha bullosa

Pneumatized turbinate bone that can widen the turbinate and narrow sinus drainage pathways.

Tina's comments:

Because I am allergic to pollens, dust, ragweed, and other airborne particles, rinsing my sinuses daily helps clean my turbinates.

28: What is Samter's triad?

Samter's triad

Also called the *aspirin triad*; comprised of aspirin allergy, asthma, and nasal polyps.

Samter's triad, also called *aspirin-induced asthma*, is a group of three diseases associated with sinusitis. This triad is comprised of nasal polyps, asthma, and aspirin sensitivity. This triad may be present in up to 10 percent of patients with asthma. The polyps in triad patients often grow to be extremely large and obstruct the nasal passageways. These polyps almost invariably regrow and will require not only surgery but close monitoring and treatment in an attempt to keep them under control. Several medical centers now offer aspirin-desensitization therapy, which may allow an aspirin-triad patient to take aspirin. This therapy also may allow the patient on aspirin after desensitization to decrease use of other medications such as oral steroids used for asthma and sinus polyps.

29: Could having sinusitis lead to having cancer?

Sinusitis as an isolated infection does not lead to cancer. However, cancers involving the sinuses can have symptoms that are very similar to sinusitis and may initially be mistaken for and treated as sinusitis. In smokers, sinus cancers are often related to exposure to chemicals that occurs over an extended period of time. Papillomas (nasal warts) of the sinuses can also be associated with cancers—but only in 10–15 percent of these patients.

PART THREE

The Doctor's Visit

When should I see a doctor for sinusitis?

What type of doctor should I see
for sinusitis?

What should I expect during the doctor's visit?

More . . .

30: When should I see a doctor for sinusitis?

When a cold or sinus symptoms persist beyond a week, it is time to see a physician. Most viral infections will resolve or at least significantly improve during that time. Acute sinusitis is readily treatable by antibiotics. If it is suspected, it should be treated to prevent the complications that may develop from a sinus infection. Symptoms that may suggest an emergency situation include significant swelling around the eye, headaches that won't go away with over-the-counter pain pills, and difficulty with vision or concentration. These may be suggestive of a sinus infection that has extended out into the eye or brain tissues.

31: What type of doctor should I see for sinusitis?

The first provider that should be consulted is a primary care doctor, nurse-practitioner, or physician assistant. They often practice in pediatrics, internal medicine, or family medicine. These providers see and manage the majority of sinus infections that develop. If sinus infections occur over and over, your primary care provider may refer you to an otolaryngologist or ENT physician for further evaluation. Additionally, if the primary care physician feels that allergies are a contributing factor, he or she may refer the patient to an allergy specialist. An **allergist** is an internal medicine physician who has completed additional training in the areas of allergy, immunology, and asthma.

Allergist

Physician who specializes in the evaluation and management of allergic disease.

If you suspect that the symptoms are urgent, you should be seen at an emergency room or urgent care clinic. Sinus infections are in the head, and there are a lot of important surrounding structures that can be affected if an infection gets out of control.

32: What should I expect during the doctor's visit?

Your primary care provider will take a history by asking you to describe your symptoms and how long you've had them. The diagnosis of sinusitis can often be made based on the history alone. However, it is important to distinguish sinusitis from other problems with similar symptoms. The doctor will ask questions about prior episodes and what therapies you have tried. Then, he or she will examine you by looking inside the nose for swelling or pus and possibly press or tap on the sinuses to check for tenderness. If appropriate, antibiotics will be prescribed. Other therapies including over-the-counter medications such as decongestants or mucus thinners may be recommended. Nasal washes and steaming the nose will help thin the infected mucus and assist with drainage.

If sinusitis recurs or the symptoms persist after appropriate therapy, your provider may order a computerized tomography scan of the sinuses. If you are referred to an otolaryngologist (an ENT doctor), he or she also will take a history and perform an examination. A nasal endoscopy, described in **Question 33**, will be performed to examine the deeper recesses of the nose.

33: What is nasal endoscopy?

An **endoscope** is a small and thin (less than the size of a pencil), rigid or flexible viewing tube with a light on one end and an eyepiece or camera attached to a video monitor on the other end. It is used to look through small holes into larger spaces. Some examples are shown in **Figure 8**. Endoscopes are used by many types of doctors to evaluate many spaces including the lungs, stomach, nose, and sinuses.

Endoscope

Thin fiberoptic rigid or flexible viewing tube with a lighted lens on one end and eyepiece on the other used to examine surfaces inside the body, such as the inside of the nose, through an orifice such as a nostril.

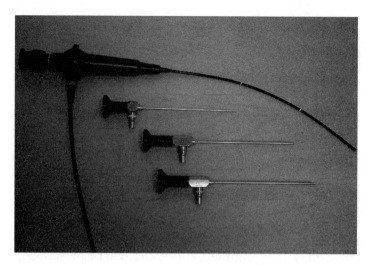

Figure 8 Nasal endoscopes

ENT doctors also use endoscopes to look at the vocal cords and other throat tissue. Nasal endoscopy is probably done in every ENT office more than 10 times each day. Before a nasal endoscopy, the staff will spray your nose with a topical decongestant to reduce the swelling and widen the path for the endoscope, and a topical anesthetic, which numbs the nose and helps decrease the chance of sneezing. The procedure is usually not painful, but some patients experience discomfort from the pressure of the endoscope. Additional numbing spray or a pediatric scope may help with such discomfort.

A nasal endoscopy allows a detailed examination of the nasal and sinus cavities.

A nasal endoscopy allows a detailed examination of the nasal and sinus cavities. During the endoscopy, the physician or other certified provider will look for areas of swelling in the mucosal membranes, for the presence of purulent secretions draining from the sinus openings, for enlargement of the turbinates, and for the presence of polyps. If pus is seen, it may be sampled to determine what organism is causing the infection.

Some doctors may allow you to see inside your nose during the endoscopy. This can be done using a TV or video monitor connected to the endoscope that you and your doctor watch. A few centers will have video glasses that the patients may wear that are connected to the endoscope, which allows them to see what it looks like inside their nose and sinuses. If you want the procedure recorded, this can often be arranged, but make sure to provide notice ahead of time because special equipment may be needed.

A nasal endoscopy is the most important diagnostic exam that an ENT will need to help with determining what may be causing sinus problems. **Figure 9** is a photo of nasal endoscopy being performed.

Tina's comments:

I like to hold on to the sides of the chair to help stabilize myself so that I remain very still during the examination. I do not want to move or twitch!

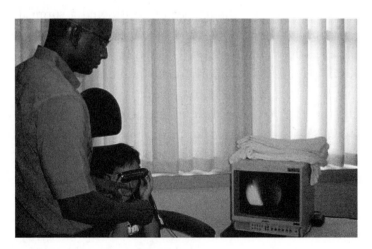

Figure 9 Nasal endoscopy being performed

Arden's comments:

I found the endoscope to cause a little discomfort, making my eyes water a little. The doctor found some pus and took a sample. The culture was positive for a staphylococcus infection and, as a result, antibiotics were prescribed. My physician provided me with a photo of what she was seeing with the endoscope—interesting, however, it was not placed in the family photo album.

Muffie's comments:

The endoscopy has never bothered me. I have never experienced pain during an exam. I enjoyed the "virtual reality" of watching the procedure!

Paula's comments:

Whenever I have a nasal endoscopy, I am confident that I am getting an accurate diagnosis. I feel no pain.

34: What are the risks of a nasal endoscopy?

A nasal endoscopy should not be considered a surgical procedure. It is a minor office-based procedure that usually takes only a few minutes. You may feel some pressure, but no pain if you are appropriately numbed by the nasal sprays. A topical nasal decongestant is typically sprayed into the nose to widen the nasal passageways, and then a topical anesthetic such as lidocaine is sprayed. Sometimes the staff may also place small cotton balls soaked in the anesthetic medication to numb the tissue further.

During the endoscopy, tell your provider if you experience significant discomfort. A "tickle" in the nose may occur even when anesthetized, so you should let the doctor know if you need to sneeze, so that he or she can remove the endoscope, which will avoid inadvertent scraping of the inside of the nose. Many doctors tell their patients to use certain words to tell them how they feel during the procedure. For instance, "ouch" and "sneeze" are common ones used so that the patient can quickly express pain or communicate pain. Try not to move without letting the doctor know so that he or she can remove the endoscope first, thus preventing any injuries.

Minor bleeding, though uncommon, could result from the procedure. This is usually due to the scope rubbing against the septum or one of the turbinates as it goes around the curves inside the nose.

35: What is a sinus culture, and what is its role in treating sinusitis?

A **culture** is taken by sampling the pus draining from the sinuses, using either a special swab or suction tube that goes into a collection device. (Some sinus culture supplies are shown in **Figure 10**.) The culture is best taken during an endoscopic examination. The specimen then is sent to the laboratory for analysis. The swab or the suction-trap container contents are cultured in the laboratory in special "food" for microorganisms such as bacteria

Culture

Obtaining a sample of infected material and sending it to the laboratory to identify causative organisms.

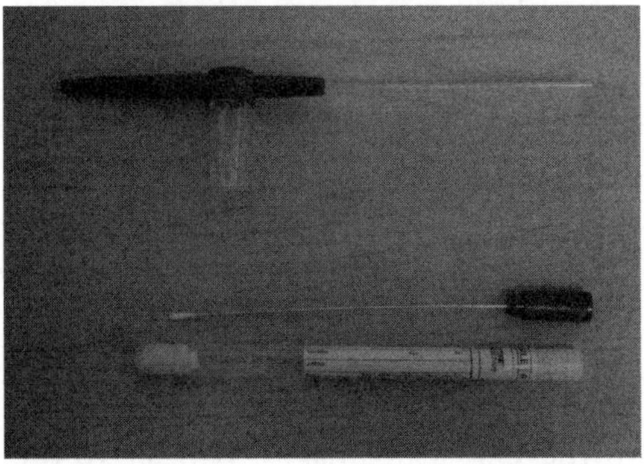

Figure 10
Sinus culture supplies

and fungi, which allows for identification of the organism causing sinusitis. The lab may also be able to determine to which antibiotics the organism is most sensitive.

After the culture results are obtained, the physician can decide which antibiotic to use if there is a bacterial infection. The culture may help to identify fungal organisms that can be found in sinus infections and help the doctor to select an antifungal medication. A negative culture may help avoid the use of unnecessary antibiotics.

36: What does a CT scan of the sinuses show?

Plain X-rays (like a basic chest X-ray) are not used much anymore in the evaluation of the sinuses. The best images of the sinuses can be obtained with a CT scan. CT scans allow the physician to examine the sinuses in detailed cross sections.

For the procedure, you lie down on the bed or platform that then slides through the CT scanner, which resembles a large donut. A typical CT scan machine is shown in **Figure 11**. Some patients may feel claustrophobic, but you are not enclosed within the machine. The scan is painless and usually quite short in length, less than 10 minutes. There are now miniature CT scanners in some doctors' offices. These allow the patient to sit on a chair during the procedure, have a less-intimidating appearance, and take only about 1 to 2 minutes to get a full sinus examination.

The interior of the sinuses, which often cannot be seen on endoscopy unless the patient has had prior surgery, can be viewed on the CT scan images. If desired, the sinuses can be imaged from more than one angle to

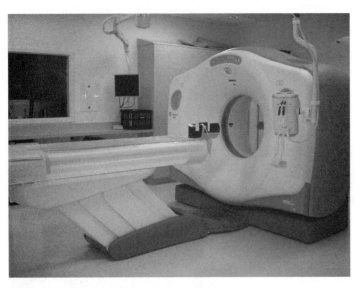

Figure 11 CT scanner

obtain images from the above, side, or front view. Cross-sectional CT images in the horizontal plane are shown in **Figure 12** and in the frontal plane in **Figure 13**. There are also office-based and operating room–based computers that can allow the extrapolation, or reconstruction of additional planar views and even create 3-D reconstructions that may allow for more detail and better surgical planning. These types of scans can be converted into **navigational scans**. The special navigational scans allow the CT-scan images to be displayed during the surgery as a global positioning-like system, which can track the location of the surgical tools inside the nose overlaid on the CT images. These types of scans can be very useful for more complex cases or in cases where prior surgery and scar tissue/disease may change the usual landmarks inside the nose.

Navigational scans

Type of CT scan performed using a specific protocol for image-guided surgery.

Arden's comments:

I complained of persistent facial pressure to my primary care physician, and he ordered a sinus CT scan. A large growth was found on the scan that eventually was removed.

45

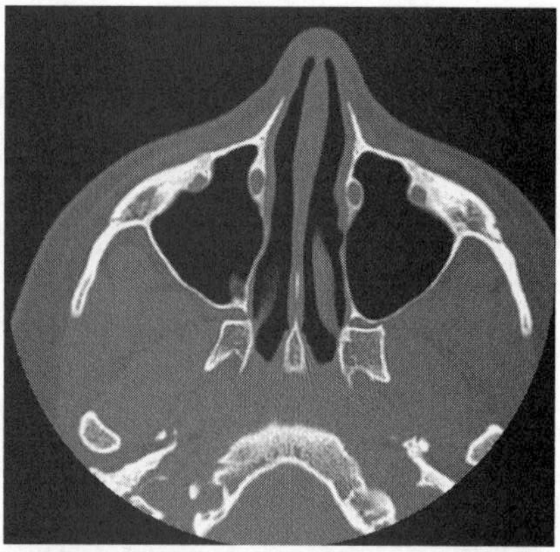

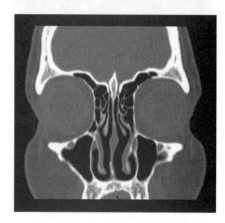

Figure 12
CT scan transverse
cross-sectional view

Figure 13
CT scan frontal
cross-sectional view

Muffie's comment:

Again, no pain, no problem!

37: What other types of studies or tests may be ordered?

Other potentially useful tests to help in the diagnosis and treatment of sinus problems may include allergy testing, nasal tissue biopsies, and immunologic blood tests. If an allergy is suspected, an allergist or ENT doctor may perform allergy testing either using skin prick tests or by getting blood tests.

If cystic fibrosis or ciliary dyskinesia (which cause defects in the tiny cilia lining the sinuses and predispose to sinus infection) is suspected, a sample of the nasal tissue can be sent for ciliary examination under the microscope. The ciliary biopsy is done by taking a small sample of the nasal mucosa under visualization of the nasal endoscopy. If an immunodeficiency (a weak immune system) is suspected, a series of blood tests may be needed to evaluate the different immune blood components that we each should have. This may require several tests to be obtained that are often done by an allergist or immunologist.

PART FOUR

Treatment of Sinusitis

What are some of the different types
of medications used to treat sinusitis?

When, how, and for how long should
I take antibiotics?

What are the risks or side effects of
taking antibiotics?

More . . .

38: What are some of the different types of medications used to treat sinusitis?

Antibiotics, steroids, decongestants, and mucus thinners may all be used in the treatment of sinusitis. There are several classes of **antibiotics**, such as penicillin, that can inhibit growth and often kill infectious bacteria, which are most often the causative organisms. Antibiotics now come in many different types that are able to treat various subcategories of bacteria. At times, a combination of antibiotics may be needed.

Antibiotics can come in liquid, chewable tablet, or pill form. Children often prefer the liquid forms because they are made with flavoring such as strawberry or bubble gum that helps with the fear of taking medicines or choking on a pill. A culture and sensitivity test (see **Question 35**) can provide helpful information to assist in the selection of the type or combination of antibiotics that will help clear a bacterial infection. However, this sinus-pus culture is reserved for patients who have failed the first- or second-line standard treatments.

Oral (by mouth) **steroids** such as prednisone or topical nasal steroids (in the form of a nasal spray or wash) may help reduce the swelling of the mucosal membranes inside the nose. They work by reducing the amount of inflammatory chemicals the body makes in the area where these medicines contact. Oral steroids go through the bloodstream and reach all the sinus walls from there. Sprays and washes are often limited to only the lower nasal tissues.

Oral steroids may help reduce the size of nasal polyps inside the sinuses. Polyps are inflamed tissue, and steroids work by shrinking back the inflammation. However, often the cause of inflammation will remain

Antibiotics, steroids, decongestants, and mucus thinners may all be used in the treatment of sinusitis.

Antibiotics

Class of medications that inhibit or kill bacterial microorganisms.

Steroids

A class of medications with strong anti-inflammatory properties.

and the polyps may regrow after the steroid pills are stopped. This is why other treatments for inflammation are continued after the steroid pills are stopped, in an attempt to decrease the chance of polyps growing back or extend the time to their recurrence.

Oral **decongestants** (like Actifed—pseudoephedrine) or topical nasal decongestants (like Afrin—oxymetalazone) also help to reduce nasal swelling. They shrink the blood vessels and swollen tissues inside the nose, the turbinates. This helps with the sense of nasal blockage that often comes with sinusitis. These medications should not be used for more than 5 days because the tissues can get used to or dependent on them. Oral decongestants can cause elevated pulse or blood pressure in some patients. Many of the medications containing decongestants are now restricted to being kept behind the counter but without a prescription because of their use in methamphetamine manufacturing. You have to ask your pharmacist for them, and he or she may record your name and the amount you purchase; there may also be limits on the amount you can purchase during a set period of time. Mucolytics such as guafenesin help to thin the thick mucus secretions and may help with the drainage into the throat.

Decongestants
Medications that shrink the lining of the nose by constricting blood vessels.

39: When, how, and for how long should I take antibiotics?

Antibiotics are prescribed when a sinus infection is not getting better by itself or with the use of simple treatments such as saline washes and over-the-counter medications. Antibiotics help when the symptoms are severe or prolonged or when there is significant concern about developing complications from sinusitis.

Antibiotics are prescribed when a sinus infection is not getting better by itself or with the use of simple treatments such as saline washes and over-the-counter medications.

Antibiotics may be given in four different ways: oral, intravenous (IV), intramuscular, or topical. Oral antibiotics are the most common form taken and are the most convenient. Most oral antibiotics are pills, but there are some antibiotics that come in liquid form. At times, the organisms present may be resistant to all of the antibiotics available in oral form. In this case, another form of delivery may be needed.

Medications may also be injected into the muscles. This is the next easiest way to get the medications, but there may be pain when it is administered as well as some muscle soreness afterward. Intramuscular medications may need to be given once a day in the doctor's office for several days.

IV medications are given through a catheter inserted in the veins of the arm. They may be administered in the hospital or at home. When used at home, a machine may be attached to the IV line that delivers the medication or a nurse may need to visit and teach the patient how to use IV medications at home.

Topical antibiotics

Form of antibiotics delivered directly to the tissues they are treating in spray, irrigation, or nebulized forms.

Nebulizer

A machine that blows the medications into a mist that is deposited on the walls of the nose and sinuses.

Topical antibiotics are also an alternative medication delivery method for certain types of patients. This form is typically reserved for patients who have already had their sinuses opened by surgery and are infected with organisms sensitive only to antibiotics that would otherwise have to be given intravenously. These topical treatments may be given in the form of home-administered washes, an office-based gel application using the endoscope, or by a nebulizer used on average twice a day at home for about 30 minutes. A **nebulizer** is a machine that blows the medications into a mist that is deposited on the walls of the nose and sinuses. Often, treatment with a nebulizer will require a significant amount of time, possibly 30–60 minutes, breathing in the medications and can be quite expensive. Many insurance companies will cover nebulized antibiotic treatment, but a few do not or will require that forms be completed by your physician's office prior to authorizing therapy.

Depending on the type of organism and how long or extensive the infection has been, the antibiotic course may be used for 5 days to several weeks. In severe cases, patients may need to stay on antibiotics for months or use various combinations to achieve the desired therapeutic effect.

40: What are the risks or side effects of taking antibiotics?

All antibiotics may have some side effects. The type of side effect will vary with the class of antibiotics used. It is important to discuss with your provider your past use of antibiotics, side effects, and problems with the different type of antibiotics that may have been prescribed. Allergic reactions may occur and range in severity from a rash to a severe response called anaphylaxis. **Anaphylaxis** is a potentially life-threatening reaction to medications when hives, throat swelling, and difficulty in breathing can occur.

Allergic reactions may occur and range in severity from a rash to a severe response called anaphylaxis.

Anaphylaxis

Life-threatening systemic allergic reaction that can cause the closure of breathing passageways.

The most common side effects of antibiotics are nausea and diarrhea. Nausea or an upset stomach can cause vomiting, which leads to the medications not having enough time to be absorbed. This can be improved if the antibiotics are taken with food. It is best if these foods are carbohydrates like bread or crackers, because proteins in meat or dairy products also can decrease the absorption of medications.

Diarrhea may be caused by alteration in the composition of the bacteria normally present in the intestines. This can often improve by eating yogurt between doses. Antibiotics can also disturb the balance of vaginal organisms, causing vaginal yeast infections in women. These can be treated with over-the-counter antifungal creams. Other antibiotics may cause sensitivity to the sun or alterations in taste. With the use of IV antibiotics, there are the additional risks of deep venous thrombosis and thrombophlebitis associated with the IV catheter. Thrombosis occurs when the veins develop a clot, and thrombophlebitis occurs when that clot subsequently becomes infected.

As with all antibiotics, medications must be carefully checked for potential drug-drug interactions

Drug-drug interactions

When one drug affects how another works.

As with all antibiotics, medications must be carefully checked for potential **drug-drug interactions**. This occurs when one drug affects how the other drug works. The way a drug is metabolized may be affected by the presence of another drug. For instance, an antibiotic could lead to another drug such as a cholesterol-lowering drug having other side effects by increasing its level in the bloodstream. In women of childbearing age, the potential or presence of a pregnancy should be evaluated because some medications can affect the fetus. If a patient is breast-feeding, certain antibiotics should be avoided because they may be transmitted through milk to the baby in concentrations that can cause side effects in the child.

Some antibiotics can cause muscle or joint problems. These can include a sore feeling in the muscles and sometimes—but rarely—tendons, especially in the heel, may rupture. It is important to call your provider if you start experiencing side effects of any sort from any medication. Most of the time these will be mild, but it is better to be safe and have your questions answered than not.

Muffie's comments:

This was where I had problems. Several antibiotics failed to work, and I experienced allergic reactions. I think the warning flags about the severity of my sinusitis should have been noticed far sooner than they were.

41: What over-the-counter medications can I use for sinusitis?

Decongestants that come in oral or topical forms are the most commonly used over-the-counter medications for sinus problems. These may include well-known medications such as Afrin or Actifed. Decongestants can improve nasal congestion and relieve the most common symptom of a sinus problem: nasal obstruction. By reducing the swelling inside the nasal cavities and sinuses, they can potentially improve sinus drainage during an infection.

Oral decongestants contain chemicals that are relatives to adrenaline. Therefore, they can be stimulants and cause the feeling of jitteriness and difficulty sleeping. Oral decongestants should be used with caution if you have high blood pressure or heart problems.

Mucus-thinning medications called **mucolytics** also may be purchased over the counter. They usually are of benefit in acute sinusitis but are often of variable benefit in chronic sinusitis. Mucolytics often make it easier to clear mucus by making it thinner. However, they can cause the volume of the mucus secretions to increase. Mucolytics may increase fertility in women of childbearing age because they thin the cervical mucus secretions, which may make it easier for sperm to cross.

Mucolytics

Medications that help to thin mucus secretions and make them easier to clear.

Over-the-counter oral antihistamines such as diphen-hydramine (Benadryl) are sometimes used for the nasal symptoms of sinusitis. However, they are often less effective than the other medications available and can even thicken and dry the mucus in the nose and sinuses. Most have the significant side effect of drowsiness, but there are nonsedating antihistamines available. They are of the most benefit for people with allergies. Other side effects are dry mouth and dry eyes, as well as problems with urinary retention for men with enlarged bladders.

Other over-the-counter medications that can improve symptoms of sinusitis include pain medications such as aspirin and other NSAIDs such as acetaminophen or ibuprofen. Preparations that combine medications from several classes, such as acetaminophen with a deconges-tant or a decongestant with a mucolytic, are also avail-able. Aspirin and other NSAIDs should be taken with caution if you have heartburn or stomach ulcers. Keep in mind that aspirin and NSAIDs will prolong the blood-clotting process and may cause you to bruise more easily.

42: What nasal sprays help sinusitis?

Nasal decongestant sprays, nasal steroid sprays, nasal antihistamines, and nasal saline sprays may be used to treat sinusitis. Nasal decongestant sprays can help to reduce the swelling of the nasal tissues during an acute sinus infection and start to work almost immediately to relieve the congestion. However, they cannot be used more than 3–5 days because excessive return of conges-tion (rebound) may occur. Rebound congestion occurs when the nasal tissues shrink in response to the decon-gestant sprays, but then return to an even more swollen state than before using the spray. This rebound congestion phenomenon is called **rhinitis medicamentosa** if it is caused by an abuse of over-the-counter topical decongestant medications.

Nasal steroid sprays may be useful in chronic sinusitis by reducing inflammation gradually. They deliver a strong concentration of steroids directly to the affected surfaces of the nasal tissues. Nasal steroid sprays should be used daily—sometimes twice a day to have any effect. They require about a week of use before they start working. They can be used safely for a long period of time but should be sprayed in an outward direction in the nose. Therefore, you should aim the bottle toward the outer corner of the eyes, because the jet of the spray can sometimes irritate the lining of the septum. This may lead to blood-tinged mucus when you blow your nose.

Rhinitis medicamentosa

Condition in which overuse of topical decongestant nasal sprays causes the lining of the nose to be nearly persistently congested due to rebound congestion.

Nasal antihistamines can help to reduce the inflammatory response of the nasal lining; they work in the same fashion as oral antihistamines except that they are only applied inside the nose, theoretically reducing the side effect profile. However, the side effects, when they occur, are similar to those of oral antihistamines. They also can cause some blood-tinged nosebleeds if used incorrectly. Nasal saline sprays help thin secretions and moisturize the nasal cavity; they can help reduce nasal congestion.

43: What are the side effects of nasal steroids?

Nasal steroids have been demonstrated to be extremely safe for long-term use, and they can be stopped and restarted without adverse effects. Oral steroids, however, cannot be used the same way. Several days are needed for

Nasal steroids have been demonstrated to be extremely safe for long-term use...

them to regain their effectiveness. The most common problems are nose bleeding and a burning sensation. If a burning sensation occurs, it may be because the formulation you are using contains alcohol as a preservative. This problem may be solved by switching to a nasal steroid in which the medications are suspended in a water solution. These are called **aqueous nasal sprays** with names like "Aqua" and "AQ." Nosebleeds occur because the medication is sprayed on the front of the nasal septum, over and over again; this will dry the area out. This can be reduced by aiming the tip of the bottle toward the outer corner of your eye on each side, which ensures that the medicine reaches the turbinates and less so toward the septum. The proper use of nasal spray bottles is demonstrated in **Figure 14**.

If nasal steroids are for the treatment of seasonal allergies, then they should be used only during allergy season, starting about 2 weeks before the allergens become a problem. Allergy doctors can test you for the allergens that you may have a problem with and also inform you of which months it is most likely to be a problem.

Aqueous nasal sprays

Nasal spray formulations that are water-based.

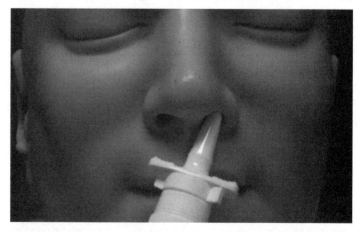

Figure 14 Proper nasal spray technique

44: What are the side effects of oral steroids?

The effects of oral steroids can be very dramatic. Often the patient will note a difference in symptoms in as little as 24 hours. Most courses of oral steroids for sinus symptoms, inflammation, or polyps are short. They are used for 5–10 days when the extent of disease or symptoms is mild. In severe cases approaching the need for surgery, longer courses may be needed.

As oral steroids enter the bloodstream and circulate throughout the body, they have a more significant side-effect profile than nasal steroids. The most common side effects caused by the short-term use of oral steroids include moodiness, irritability, stomach upset, and weight gain. Acne, fluid retention, and thinning of the skin with easy bruising may also occur with use. Long-term use can lead to abnormal fat deposits, developing cataracts, blood pressure problems, and osteoporosis (weakened bones).

Use of oral steroids for more than 1 or 2 weeks can suppress the body's ability to make its own steroids, such as cortisol. This is a hormone that helps your body respond to stress. Longer courses of steroids can make the body more susceptible to infections. Gradually reducing the steroid dose during a cycle of steroid treatment allows the body time to adjust by slowly increasing its natural cortisol production. Steroid use can cause heartburn, indigestion, or in rare cases, stomach ulcers and gastric bleeding. These may occur when longer courses of these medications are used. Using acid-reducing and stomach-protective medications such as Zantac or Pepcid may help reduce the chance of these problems occurring.

Paula's comments:

Long courses of steroids can really affect your life. Unless absolutely necessary, I would discourage their use. While taking them, I never slept, gained lots of weight, and I was often emotional ... I cried a lot.

45: What are nasal saline irrigations, and how are they performed?

Nasal saline irrigation or *lavage* is essentially a nasal douche with a salt solution balanced with baking soda so that it will not sting. These irrigations are easy, inexpensive, and quite effective at improving many of the common symptoms associated with nasal and sinus problems. Because there are really no negative side effects, they can be performed as often as desired.

Nasal saline irrigation

Flushing the nose with a large volume of salt solution

The saline rinses help to flush out excess mucus and other unwanted debris that can irritate the tissue lining the nose and sinuses and cause inflammation. Syringes, special bottles, or neti pots, which look like small teapots, may all be used to perform the irrigation. Examples of a syringe, squeeze bottle, and a neti pot are shown in **Figure 15**. Regardless of which device you use, it is important to keep it clean.

The saline rinses help to flush out excess mucus and other unwanted debris that can irritate the tissue lining the nose and sinuses and cause inflammation.

Though it is preferred to use boiled or distilled water, regular tap water is usually clean enough for nasal irrigation. Make sure that if you are using well water there is a purification system used to decrease fungal elements. Kosher salt or sea salt is often a purer form and has less sugars and chemicals than regular table salt. In a pinch, regular table salt can also be used. Regular

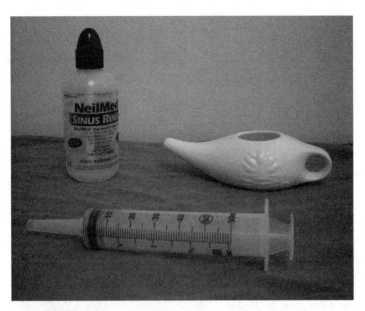

Figure 15 Nasal irrigation supplies

baking soda is used to balance the pH of the solution so that it is less likely to sting. In addition, there are pre-mixed salt and baking soda packages that may be used to make saline solution. Nasal saline irrigation solution can be made with 2–3 heaping tablespoons of kosher or sea salt and 1 teaspoon of baking soda dissolved into 1 liter of distilled water.

Saline irrigations are performed by flushing a syringe-full or half a bottle or pot of the saline solution through each nasal cavity while standing with your head over the sink or in the shower. Syringes or squeeze bottles allow irriga-tion with more force, while a neti pot allows passive flow of liquid into the nose. It is not necessary to inhale while irrigating; the water may drain out the nose on the same or the other side or the mouth. **Figure 16** demonstrates nasal irrigation with a specially designed squeeze bottle.

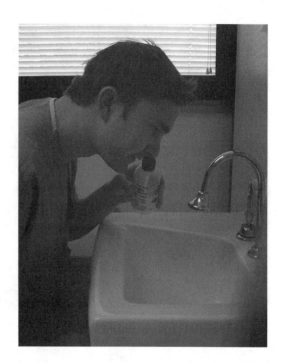

Figure 16
Nasal irrigation
demonstration

Most people perform nasal saline irrigations twice a day, but they can be performed more often. It is recommended after surgery to help clear the sinuses of old blood but should only be started when the surgeon says it is okay.

Motorized devices such as the Grossan or Waterpik irrigators may be used to irrigate the nose. However, the water is often more forceful than other irrigation devices and could cause bleeding if used too early after surgery. This additional force may be useful for a few patients who have thick crusts but is probably not necessary for routine irrigations. It is also important to examine these devices frequently because mold may grow inside, where it is dark and damp. The plastic containers or tubing also can serve as a medium on which bacteria can grow. For this reason, those using the irrigation devices should clean them often or use devices that are inexpensive and can be replaced monthly or after an infection.

Tina's comments:

I always thought a saline irrigation in my nose would be a very unpleasant experience. To my great surprise, it actually felt good to flush the stuff out of my nose. It helps to warm the irrigating solution to at least room temperature or a little warmer.

Paula's comments:

Nasal irrigations help. You can rinse with saline as needed.

46: Are there medications that can be added to the nasal irrigations?

Steroids, antifungals, and antibiotics can all be added to saline solution to treat different subtypes of sinusitis. These topical medication washes can be used to treat infections with antibiotics or antifungals that may have otherwise needed to be treated with pills or IV medications. When given topically, the side effect profile is much less severe because exposure to the medication is limited to the affected areas. Topical medications also do not linger in the bloodstream as when given in the oral or IV forms. Those taking them in this manner do not run the risk of causing other side effects in nonsinus tissues.

47: Are topical antibiotics right for me?

Nasal antibiotic sprays, antibiotic irrigations, and nebulizers (machines that turn the medication into a fine mist that is inhaled to allow spreading of the medication on the lining of the nose) are all forms of topical antibiotics. Various medications can be compounded by a specialized pharmacist into a liquid form to be sprayed or washed into the nose or delivered through a nebulizer. Medications also can be mixed into nasal irrigation solutions so that the lining of the nasal cavities can be bathed in the medication. Topical medications are particularly useful in patients whose sinuses have been opened by sinus surgery and continue to have infections, swelling, or symptoms.

48: What are some complications of untreated acute sinusitis?

Sinus infections may extend from the sinuses to other structures. **Preseptal cellulitis** develops when sinus infections extend to the skin and soft tissue surrounding the eye. In addition to the symptoms of sinusitis, the skin around the eye becomes red and puffy, and the patient may have trouble opening the eyelid.

When the infection extends to the bone within the orbit or the eye socket, it becomes a **subperiosteal** (below bony layers) **abscess**. If a collection of infected pus develops within the fat or muscles of the eye socket, it is called an **orbital abscess**. When the infection extends into the eye socket, the patient may have problems moving the eye, have pain within the eye, or the eye may protrude from the face.

Cavernous sinus thrombosis occurs when the sinus infection extends into the blood vessels behind the sphenoid sinus. All these infections must be treated with antibiotics. Preseptal cellulitis is often treatable by antibiotics alone, but the others require surgical therapy to drain the sinuses. Sinus infections can sometimes extend into the brain tissue by direct erosion through the bone that separates them. Patients with extension into the brain will often have changes in their mental status or their level of consciousness.

Sinus infections may extend from the sinuses to other structures.

Preseptal cellulitis

Complication of sinusitis that develops when sinus infections extend to the skin and soft tissue surrounding the eye.

Subperiosteal abscess

Complication of sinusitis in which infection of the skin around the eye spreads to the bone within the eye socket.

Orbital abscess

Complication of sinusitis in which a collection of infected pus develops within the fat or muscles of the eye socket.

Cavernous sinus thrombosis

Complication of sinusitis that occurs when the sinus infection extends into the blood vessels behind the sphenoid sinus.

49: What are complications of untreated chronic sinusitis?

Erosion or thinning of the bone between the brain and the sinuses or the eyes and the sinuses can occur if a sinus infection is prolonged. With the development of sinus polyps or mucus-filled cysts, they can expand within the sinuses and apply pressure to the surrounding areas. Blocked sinuses will continue to form mucus that can enlarge to become a **mucocoele**, which is a mucus-filled cyst. A mucocoele can cause headaches, or if it displaces the eye in the eye socket, it can cause double vision. The formation of a mucocoele is shown in a CT scan of a sinus in **Figure 17**.

Mucocoele
Mucus-filled collection.

Sinus infections can also extend into the face and down into the teeth or gums. At times, especially in patients with immune system problems, sinus infections may spread bacteria into the bloodstream and cause sepsis, which is a systemic blood-borne infection associated with high fevers and even renal failure.

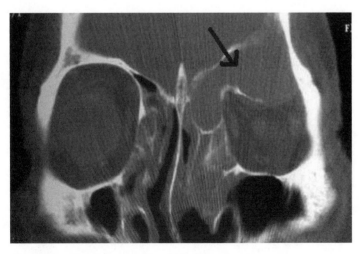

Figure 17 Orbital complication of sinusitis

50: When is sinus surgery necessary?

When the complications of sinusitis given earlier develop, sinus surgery may be needed on an urgent basis. Less-urgent sinus surgery may be necessary when chronic sinusitis fails to respond to extensive and thorough medical therapy. This is often called **maximal medical therapy**. For chronic sinusitis, this usually involves a prolonged antibiotic course, preferably based on the results of a culture, a course of steroids, nasal saline irrigations, and if allergy is identified, treatment for allergies.

Maximal medical therapy

Using the most extensive courses and optimal combinations of medications possible for treatment.

CT scans also are needed to confirm that symptoms are related to the sinuses. As an example, a patient with headache as a "sinus" symptom may have other causes for such (e.g., migraine or tension/stress headaches) that would not respond to sinus surgery. An endoscopy will be used to help determine the causative agents and potential treatment options for them.

PART FIVE

Sinus Surgery

What is functional endoscopic sinus
surgery (FESS)? Who will benefit from it?
What are its advantages?

How many sinus surgeries are performed
each year in the United States?

What happens during sinus surgery?

More . . .

51: What is functional endoscopic sinus surgery (FESS)? Who will benefit from it? What are its advantages?

FESS represents a significant advance compared to the open sinus procedures...

Functional endoscopic sinus surgery (FESS)

Minimally invasive form of sinus surgery that attempts to restore normal sinus drainage pathways.

Nasal packing

Sponge-like or ribbon-like material placed in the nose to help stop bleeding.

In the late 1980s and early 1990s, a minimally invasive approach to surgery for sinusitis called **functional endoscopic sinus surgery** (FESS) evolved. FESS represents a significant advance compared to the open sinus procedures performed prior to the development of FESS. The goal of FESS is to reestablish physiologically normal sinus drainage pathways by removing or correcting diseased pieces of tissues in key areas of sinus obstruction. Small rigid telescopes, called endoscopes, are inserted into the nose, and the surgery is performed using fine instruments to open the sinuses. The operating room set-up for FESS is shown in **Figure 18**, and **Figure 19** is an image from a video monitor showing FESS in progress.

There are several advantages to FESS over the open sinus procedures that preceded it. To begin with, the ability to see within the nose and sinuses is much improved. Before endoscopes were used, surgeons mostly made incisions in order to directly access the interior of the affected sinus. Procedures that could be done from within the nose were illuminated with headlights, which are special lamps that are suspended from the surgeon's forehead; this limited the view.

Open sinus procedures often required facial incisions with resulting visible scars and lots of **nasal packing**. The open procedures were more likely to cause facial or eye bruising and swelling. With FESS, there are usually no visible signs that surgery has been performed because the surgery is almost always done completely through the nostrils. Recovery is usually faster and there is usually less postoperative pain and bleeding. Nasal packing, described later in **Question 65**, is used infrequently in FESS.

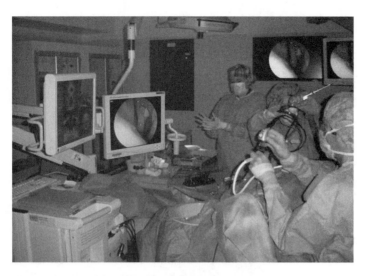

Figure 18 Operating room set-up for sinus surgery

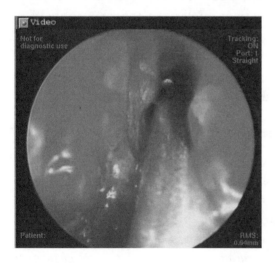

Figure 19
View of video
monitor during
sinus surgery

When patients with sinusitis do not improve after
repeated courses of antibiotics and reasonable trials of
the other medications used to treat sinusitis, the otolaryngologist may recommend undergoing FESS. The
recommendation will be based on the physical examination, nasal endoscopy, and CT scan findings. The
decision to perform surgery should be made only after
carefully considering the risks and benefits.

Age is not usually a major factor in decision making for or against sinus surgery. Being an older surgery candidate is not usually a problem, especially if the patient is otherwise healthy. It is important, however, to determine if the majority of the problematic symptoms are attributable to sinus disease and not to allergic rhinitis. Patients with poorly managed allergic rhinitis in the absence of sinus disease will not benefit from sinus surgery.

Patient preferences also play a role in the decision. For instance, some patients may prefer partial relief of symptoms from repeated courses of antibiotics for recurrent sinusitis to undergoing surgery. However, eventually, most patients who take antibiotics frequently develop infections from antibiotic-resistant organisms or develop a serious reaction to or intolerance of certain antibiotics. The decision to have sinus surgery is usually made by patients when the impact of the sinusitis on their quality of life is so significant that a successful surgery can improve their ability to function in daily life.

Arden's comments:

I have undergone two FESS procedures, one with an image guidance system. My surgeries were performed on an outpatient basis and recovery was quick and uneventful. The first FESS was to remove a large polyp and correct a deviated septum. The polyp was determined to be an inverted papilloma, a type of noncancerous tumor, so the second surgery was done to remove additional affected tissue.

52: How many sinus surgeries are performed each year in the United States?

Approximately 538,000 sinus surgeries were performed in 1995 in the United States, according to the Sinus and Allergy Health Partnership. It is one of the most common procedures done by ENT doctors. Sinus surgeries can be done in either free-standing ambulatory surgery centers or in hospital operating rooms. Most FESS is performed as an outpatient procedure, which is sometimes also referred to as same-day surgery.

53: What happens during sinus surgery?

FESS can be performed under either local or **general anesthesia**. Factors that will be taken into consideration when selecting the anesthetic type are the extensiveness of surgery and the relative anesthetic risk factors present in the patient for surgery. Most people have the procedure performed under general anesthesia.

Small rigid telescopes (nasal endoscopes) are attached to cameras. The cameras are in turn attached to video monitors so that the surgeon can see the deeper recesses of the nose and then into the sinuses when they are opened. Various fine cutting instruments and special tissue "shavers" called **microdebriders** are used to remove diseased tissue. Polyps are removed from the nasal cavity. The sinus openings are identified, opened, and widened by removing the diseased bone and mucosa blocking the ostia. Clearing the sinus openings can be best analogized to imagining that the sinuses are a room and that sinus openings are a door; sinus surgery involves completely removing the door to the room.

A special computer navigation system, or **image-guidance system**, may also be used during the surgery to assist the surgeon in confirming the location of certain structures during the surgery. These systems can help surgeons in situations where the anatomy of the nose and sinuses is complex or altered by previous surgery. The "map" for the navigation system is a CT scan done prior to the surgery.

Most people have the procedure performed under general anesthesia.

General anesthesia

Form of anesthesia in which the patient is completely asleep and breathing is assisted by a ventilator.

Microdebriders

Sinus surgery instrument that sucks tissue into it and removes the tissue with a spinning blade.

Image-guidance system

Computer navigation system for surgery that helps provide the surgeon with additional anatomical information.

At the end of the procedure and depending on the amount of bleeding present, nasal packing made of an absorbent material may possibly be used. Patients are then taken to the recovery room. For the final step, the removed tissue is routinely sent to a pathologist for analysis.

Paula's comments:

I had no complications and very little discomfort after my surgeries. My only concern was that I might have an asthma attack.

54: What are the risks of sinus surgery?

Both major and minor risks are associated with FESS, but the minor complications are more common than major ones. Minor risks associated with sinus surgery during the immediate postoperative period include bleeding, pain/discomfort, congestion, and infection. Nose bleeding is common after surgery, especially during the first 24 to 48 hours after surgery. Pain, congestion, and discomfort may be present due to the manipulation of the endoscopes and instruments within the nasal cavities. Infections can develop during the postoperative period because the old blood and mucus can pool in the sinuses after surgery, serving as a nutrient source for bacteria if they remain there too long.

A minor risk that can occur a longer period of time after surgery is the development of scar tissue. Scar tissue formation is a significant cause for the failure of sinus surgery because it can close off the opened sinuses, causing infections to recur. Scar tissue can often be prevented with meticulous tissue handling during surgery and aggressive cleaning of the nasal cavities after surgery. The possibility that additional surgeries may be required because the disease redevelops should be considered as a risk of surgery.

Because the sinuses are located close to the **orbit** (eye socket) and the brain, there are major risks of injury to the eye and the brain during sinus surgery. Injuries to the eye and brain are extremely rare during sinus surgery but can be devastating. Major risks include a cerebrospinal (brain) fluid leak, meningitis, and brain injury. **Cerebrospinal fluid (CSF) leaks,** leakage of the fluid surrounding the brain, can occur when the bone between the sinuses and the brain is absent or injured and then the dura, which is the tough covering of the brain, is violated. CSF leaks are more likely to occur when the ethmoid sinuses are operated on but also occur during procedures on the frontal and sphenoid sinuses. If these leaks occur, they generally are identified during the procedure and often can be repaired during the procedure endoscopically with a patch of tissue from the lining of the nose or the cartilage from the septum. Less often, a neurosurgeon may be consulted to assist with repair of the CSF leak.

Meningitis can occur if the tissue covering the brain, the meninges, is violated and infection or inflammation of that tissue develops. Meningitis is treated with antibiotics. Direct brain injury can occur if the bone and the tissue covering the brain are cut through and the brain is entered with an instrument. Direct brain injury will require consultation with a neurosurgeon.

Several types of eye complications are possible. These include developing watery eyes due to tear duct injury or double vision due to eye muscle injury when the eye socket is inadvertently entered. Blindness can occur if there is injury to the **optic nerve**, which is responsible for vision, or if there is bleeding within the eye socket that damages the optic nerve due to increased pressure and blockage of blood flow. Tear duct injury often can

Because the sinuses are located close to the orbit (eye socket) and the brain, there are major risks of injury to the eye and the brain during sinus surgery.

Orbit
Eye socket and its contents.

Cerebrospinal fluid (CSF) leak
Leakage of the fluid that the brain normally floats within.

Meningitis
Infection of the tissues that cover and surround the brain.

Optic nerve
Nerve that transmits signals from the eye to the brain.

be corrected with another procedure. Although difficult, it is also possible to surgically correct injury to the muscles moving the eye. Unfortunately, injury to the optic nerve cannot be repaired. Complications involving the eye will usually be managed with the assistance of an ophthalmologist or eye specialist.

Risks to the brain, heart, kidneys, and liver from general anesthesia should also be carefully weighed. Although uncommon, it is possible to have a stroke or heart attack while under general anesthesia or during the postoperative period because blood flow may be altered during anesthesia. Furthermore, the body can be stressed by the surgery itself, precipitating a heart attack. In addition, there are rare reactions to anesthetic medications, such as **malignant hyperthermia**, that can be life threatening. Malignant hyperthermia is a condition in which a patient responds to a certain anesthetic medication by developing a high fever that can lead to cardiovascular collapse. Careful preoperative consultation with an anesthesiologist should allow the identification of most anesthetic risks for a particular patient.

Malignant hyperthermia

Life-threatening high body temperature and muscle rigidity in response to certain anesthetic medications; runs in families.

55: What can I do to reduce the risk of complications?

Sinus surgery should be performed by an experienced physician who has performed a significant number of the procedures recently. Careful preoperative planning and meticulous surgery will reduce the risk of complications. Following postoperative care instructions carefully and keeping postoperative exam appointments also will help the physician monitor your progress. Taking the medications prescribed by your physician after surgery will help you recover from surgery. Irrigating your

Sinus surgery should be performed by an experienced physician who has performed a significant number of the procedures recently.

nose will help clear out old blood and mucus, preventing an infection and promoting wound healing. You should immediately notify your physician if anything unusual develops after surgery, such as protracted bleeding or changes in your vision.

Based upon your age, different blood tests, X-rays, and electrocardiograms may be ordered as part of your preoperative testing. These tests are requested to look for possible problems such as anemia or problems clotting blood. You and your physician will review your medical history carefully and determine if you need additional evaluation by other physicians prior to undergoing surgery. For instance, if you have had chest pain that has never been evaluated, this should probably be worked up prior to the surgery since the surgery or anesthesia can precipitate a heart attack. You should also check with your primary care physician to find out if there are any changes to your medications or if there are problems that need to be addressed prior to undergoing general anesthesia.

If you have a personal history of easy bruising, prolonged bleeding, or problems with anesthetics, you should notify your physician so that these problems may be monitored with diagnostic testing and arrangements made for management or prevention of these problems prior to surgery. Both bleeding disorders and life-threatening anesthesia medication reactions can run in families, so you should also check with immediate family members to find out if they have had difficulty with prolonged bleeding or anesthetic complications during their procedures.

Aspirin and other NSAIDs (ibuprofen, naproxen) need to be stopped 1 week prior to surgery to avoid excessive bleeding. Supplements such as gingko, ginger, ginseng, and garlic can also prolong bleeding times. Vitamin E can also contribute to bleeding. All prescription and nonprescription medications should be disclosed to your physicians and nurses.

56: What is image-guided sinus surgery, and how does it work?

Image-guided systems are essentially like global positioning satellite (GPS) systems for the anatomy of your head.

Image-guided systems are essentially like global positioning satellite (GPS) systems for the anatomy of your head. These systems are used to aid the surgeon in confirming the location and proximity of critical structures like the thin bone that separates the contents of the eye socket from the ethmoid sinuses when the interior of the nose and sinuses is distorted by unusual anatomy or prior surgery. Assistance from image-guidance technology is especially useful during surgery on the frontal and sphenoid sinuses, when the adjacent brain and eyes are at risk of injury.

Using the GPS analogy to explain image-guided navigation for sinus surgery, GPS navigation requires a map, satellites surrounding the planet, the tracked vehicle, and a computer in the vehicle programmed to integrate the information. To use the image-guidance navigation system, the "map," a CT scan of the sinuses, is performed using a specific navigation system protocol. For many systems, a special mask or markers are placed on your face during the scan to serve as reference points. When the surgeon plans to use anatomical features such as the corner of your eye, the front of the ear, or the bridge of the nose as reference points, the scan is done without markers or a mask. The CT scan is transferred to a disk, which is then loaded into the image-guidance computer.

During surgery, the patient's head is the "planet" and either a detection array or a mask serves as the "satellites" surrounding the head. The CT scan images loaded into the system are then calibrated to the patient's anatomy using preset reference points, which may be the mask, markers, or specific anatomic points on the face. The position of the sinus surgery instrument, or "vehicle," can then be tracked by the computer by integrating the information detected from the satellites and the vehicle and comparing it to the information on the CT scan "map."

Two types of sinus surgery image-guidance systems exist: one is based on an electromagnetic field and the other on optical tracking using infrared light. Both types are similar in accuracy and widely used in operating rooms. The selection of a particular system depends on the preferences of the surgeon and the facility. **Figure 20** shows an image-guided surgery system, and **Figure 21** shows the views seen on an image-guidance monitor during surgery.

Arden's comments:

Since I had had a prior FESS surgical procedure to remove an inverted papilloma polyp, I was a candidate for a second FESS procedure with image guidance to remove all of the inverted papilloma tissue in my sinus. Just prior to my surgical procedure, the surgeon placed marker stickers on my face and neck. I was then taken to the radiology department for a CT scan, which was recorded on a cassette. The cassette and I then proceeded to the operating room equipped with the image-guidance system.

I fully embraced this technology after watching a video of an actual image-guided procedure on the Internet. I felt much more comfortable about the potential complications due to the close proximity of the brain and the optic nerve. With the image-guided sinus surgery, the surgeon can "see," with a high degree of accuracy, the orientation of the endoscope and surgical instruments relative to the anatomical structures shown on the CT scan.

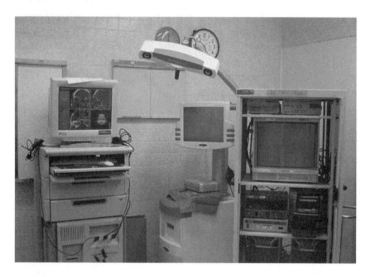

Figure 20 Image-guided surgery system

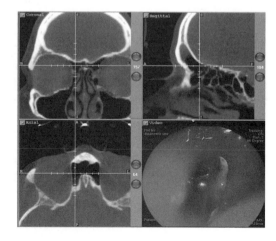

Figure 21
View of image-
guidance
system screen
during surgery

57: When is image-guidance needed during sinus surgery?

Although the use of image-guidance systems is increasing in endoscopic sinus surgery, it is not required for all sinus procedures. Image-guided surgical navigation is not a substitute for sound surgical judgment and operative experience. Though it is tempting to demand its use during every surgery, its use does not make much of a difference in sinuses that have not been operated on before. Cases with straightforward anatomy also do not require image-guidance. Furthermore, when they are not indicated, the use of an image-guidance system unnecessarily adds to the length of the procedure and possibly the cost of the procedure.

Image-guided surgical navigation is not a substitute for sound surgical judgment and operative experience.

Image guidance is most useful while operating on patients who have had previous sinus surgery, patients who have more complicated anatomy of the frontal or sphenoid sinuses, cases of benign tumor growths such as inverted papilloma, and patients who have thinning of the bone between the sinuses and the brain or the eye. If the site of a CSF leak is identified on a preoperative CT scan, the image-guidance system may also be useful during CSF leak repairs to help isolate the bony defect to be patched. In some cases in which both bony and soft-tissue detail is important, special technology to merge CT scans, which provide good bony detail, and magnetic resonance imaging (MRI), which offers better soft tissue detail, can be merged to take advantage of both views during the surgery.

One thing that image guidance does not do is show your surgeon what has already been removed during the surgery. Real-time imaging during sinus surgery is not possible at this time, though both surgeons and the manufacturers of the image-guidance systems certainly hope that it can be developed in the future.

58: What is the success rate of sinus surgery?

In studies, success rates for FESS cited in medical journals range from 60–95 percent. Most studies lump patients with varying levels of severity of sinusitis together, which may make the results from them difficult to generalize to other patients. Furthermore, studies in the medical journals often define "success" differently. Most studies look at results about 1 year after surgery, which should be kept in mind when interpreting the results. Many patients do well after sinus surgery in both subjective outcomes from patient surveys and from objective data obtained from postoperative endoscopic exam and CT scans.

The symptoms that respond best to sinus surgery are facial pressure and nasal obstruction. The sense of smell can sometimes be worse after surgery, and it usually requires a long period of time to recover. Postnasal drainage and cough due to the post-nasal drainage may not improve for a long time until the inflammation of the mucosa in the sinuses has resolved; it may not even change because the production of mucus is part of normal nasal function and is also tied to the inflammation from allergic or sensitivity responses. Because the sinus drainage pathways are more open after sinus surgery, drainage from the nose may sometimes even increase.

Success rates also will vary depending on the amount of sinus disease and the length of time that it has been present. Disease that is limited in extent has a higher degree of success; for instance, a patient with chronic sinusitis in just one maxillary sinus will generally have more long-term improvement than someone in whom all eight sinuses are affected. Sinus surgeries for nasal polyps have success rates in the 60 percent range because polyps frequently redevelop and the patients will need to have additional surgeries. Patients with nasal polyps and Samter's triad or CF further increase the likelihood of recurrence and negatively impact success rates.

59: Could rhinoplasty/septoplasty/ turbinate reduction be done at the same time as my sinus surgery?

Septoplasty and **turbinate reduction** can be combined with sinus surgery if the procedures are needed to improve access to the nasal cavity or to improve airflow inside the nasal cavity by widening the nasal cavity. These procedures are commonly performed together. The advisability of combining cosmetic **rhinoplasty** and sinus surgery will vary based upon the personal opinions and experiences of your physician or physicians.

The benefits and risks of having both surgeries done at the same time should be discussed with your physician. For instance, undergoing anesthesia only once and thus only missing work once would be the advantage of performing them together. Postoperative complication rates are not higher when the procedures are done together. However, the surgical and therefore anesthetic time will be prolonged, which may increase the anesthetic risks in patients with co-morbid conditions.

There may be conflicting priorities with combining the procedures. For instance, although uncommon, if a large amount of nasal packing is needed for bleeding from the sinus surgery, it could disrupt achievement of the desired aesthetic effect of the rhinoplasty. If either the rhinoplasty or FESS is complicated, it is usually preferable to perform rhinoplasty and sinus surgery separately.

Septoplasty

Surgery to correct the crooked areas of the nasal septum.

Turbinate reduction

Surgery to reduce the size of the inferior turbinates.

Rhinoplasty

Cosmetic surgery to alter the external appearance of the nose.

60: How do I select a doctor to do the surgery?

Your primary care physician will refer you to a surgeon he or she is are familiar with and respect and trust to manage your disease. The local and state medical societies also keep lists or directories of physicians in their regions. In addition, there are listings of board-certified otolaryngologists on several Web sites, which are included in the appendix at the end of the book. Local magazines may also publish "best doctor" lists that you can consult. Other people with sinus problems may be a good resource.

Important factors to take into account when selecting a surgeon are the amount of experience they have performing the surgery, how often they perform the surgery, and the rapport they establish with you.

Important factors to take into account when selecting a surgeon are the amount of experience they have performing the surgery, how often they perform the surgery, and the rapport they establish with you. If you have already had sinus surgery and the problem has returned or gotten worse, you may wish to seek out the opinion of an otolaryngologist who has additional training in the subspecialty of rhinology. Though there are relatively few fellowship-trained specialists in rhinology, they can usually be found in larger cities and in university medical centers.

61: Do I have to have sinus surgery right away or can it wait? Will my insurance pay for it?

Sinus surgery is only an emergency when there are complications that threaten vision or may cause brain infection. The sinuses must be opened and drained immediately in these cases because the source of the infection must be treated. The majority of sinus surgeries in the United States are done on an elective basis. There should be adequate time to allow planning of any required preoperative diagnostic testing and medical evaluations needed and to allow the patient to make arrangements to take time off work. Sinus surgery, exclusive of sinusitis with eye or brain complications, should be undertaken only when all reasonable nonsurgical options have been exhausted.

The most important reason to decide to have sinus surgery is how the symptoms of sinusitis are making you feel. Most cases of chronic sinusitis that do not respond to medical therapy will typically worsen over time and become more symptomatic. It is important to remember that there is no cure for sinusitis and to have realistic expectations for the outcome of surgery; sinus surgery is unlikely to completely eliminate all sinusitis symptoms, and some medications will still be necessary.

If you have tried the different medications for sinusitis and still have disease based upon your symptoms, your physician's physical and endoscopic examination, and on a CT scan, your insurance company will most likely cover the procedure as a medical necessity. Medications needed after surgery should also be covered. It is important to carefully review the benefits included in your medical insurance coverage in order to determine what portion of the costs is covered. The portion of the costs you are responsible for includes the co-pays for the procedures; if you have a deductible, you need to know how much of your deductible you have met because that will also impact how much you pay.

You should also check if the surgeon, the anesthesiologist, and the surgical facility are considered in your network or out of your insurance network because the reimbursement will be less or possibly nonexistent if you are considered out of network by your health plan. Your doctor's office and the financial or billing office at the facility where you are having the surgery done can give you an estimate of your expected out-of-pocket costs, but the final bill may be different than that estimate.

62: What should I expect the day of surgery?

In preparation for general anesthesia, you should not eat or drink after midnight the day before. This is done to reduce the risk of aspiration during intubation for general anesthesia, which is the insertion of a breathing tube. Aspiration occurs when stomach contents are unintentionally sucked into the lungs, and can cause aspiration pneumonia.

Consultation with the anesthesiologist usually will take place prior to the day of surgery, either during a presurgical screening appointment or a telephone call. During that visit, the anesthesiologist or the surgery center nurses often will advise you regarding which of your regular medications to take before surgery or if you need to adjust the dosage of the medications. In general, essential medications such as those for heart disease and high blood pressure are to be taken with small sips of water. Medications for diabetes will be either held or reduced in dose, because there is no food to elevate the blood sugar level.

You should dress comfortably and minimize the amount of valuables you carry to the surgery center or the hospital. The surgery center or hospital will call the day before the surgery to tell you what time you need to arrive, usually 1 to 2 hours before the surgery start time.

In preparation for general anesthesia, you should not eat or drink after midnight the day before.

Once there, you will check in at the admitting office. The admitting office will then send you to the "holding" area, where you will wait prior to going into surgery.

Once you are in the holding area or preoperative area, you will change into a hospital gown in the dressing room. The nurses then perform their preoperative nursing assessment by taking your vital signs and reviewing your medical history and list of medications. Then, the nurse will probably start an IV line to begin hydrating you. When the nurse, the anesthesiologist, and the surgeon have all seen you and the anesthetic and operating room staff have finished preparing the equipment and the instruments, you will be taken to the operating room. Depending on the setting, you may walk in yourself with a healthcare provider escort or you may be wheeled into the room in a wheelchair or on a gurney.

The length of time the surgery will take depends on several factors. It will vary according to the number of sinuses that need to be opened during the surgery, the severity of the inflammation, the number of nasal polyps, the presence of scarring, and the amount of bleeding encountered during the procedure. Most sinus surgeries last between 1 and 3 hours. As FESS techniques have been refined, surgical times have lengthened due to the more meticulous dissection techniques involved. If at any time, the surgeon feels that it is unsafe to proceed, he or she will stop the surgery.

63: What should I expect after surgery?

After surgery is complete, you will be taken to the recovery room, where the nurses and doctors will make sure you are stable prior to going home or being transferred to a hospital room. The majority of sinus surgery performed

The majority of sinus surgery performed in the United States is done as a same-day surgery...

in the United States is done as a same-day surgery so you will spend 1 to 4 hours in the recovery room after surgery. Most people do not remember the early period in the recovery room since the effects of the anesthetic medications as well as the pain medications are still in place. Before you are discharged, the staff will usually make sure that you are sufficiently alert, able to tolerate liquids, and able to urinate.

If you had general anesthesia, you may continue to feel nausea for the rest of the day and possibly the next day.

If you had general anesthesia, you may continue to feel nausea for the rest of the day and possibly the next day. Self-limited nosebleeds or bloody mucus drainage are common after FESS, particularly during the 48 hours; it may continue for up to a week after surgery. A "mustache"-type dressing that sits under your nose, shown in **Figure 22**, will help catch fluids draining from the nose and help avoid soiling of clothing.

Nasal congestion and stuffiness are also expected after sinus surgery due to swelling of the nasal mucosa and the mucus drainage. Topical decongestants such as oxymetazoline (Afrin) can help with the stuffiness. Avoid blowing your nose during this time. Nasal irrigations usually begin the day after surgery. They should be performed twice a day. Consistent irrigation will help the healing process by clearing out accumulated old blood and mucus.

A dull headache may develop and will be relieved with pain medications, which your physician will prescribe for you; sleeping with your head elevated on several pillows may also help. Depending on the condition of your sinuses, you may also be given antibiotics and/or oral steroids after FESS.

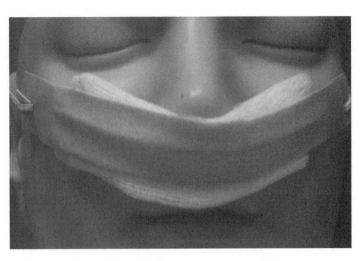

Figure 22 "Mustache"-style dressing

You may resume eating and drinking whatever you like after surgery. It is important to make sure you drink enough liquids to prevent dehydration. You can resume driving a day or two after surgery but should not drive when you are taking narcotic pain medications. Aspirin and other NSAIDs should be held for another week after surgery, if possible, to decrease the risk of bleeding. Nasal steroid sprays and antihistamines should also be held for a week after surgery.

64: When can I go back to work after sinus surgery?

Most people take about a week off work to recover from surgery, but the amount of time you should take off will vary according to the type of work you do. For the first week after surgery, a significant amount of fatigue is expected and is a normal part of the recovery process. Most people will tire more quickly than usual even

Most people take about a week off work to recover from surgery...

87

while performing light activities. The majority of people will feel that they are close to "returned to normal" after about 2 weeks.

Strenuous activity such as heavy lifting or running should be avoided for 2 weeks after surgery because it may promote bleeding. You should plan events at work and in your personal life accordingly. If you work at a desk, then a week off should be fine; however, if your works involves heavy manual labor, then 10 to 14 days off work would be more appropriate.

65: What is nasal packing?

Nasal packing is a long strip of gauze or a finger-shaped sponge that is put into the nasal cavity to apply direct pressure, absorb blood, and help stop bleeding in the nose. Some nasal packings are made with materials that can help blood clot or keep the tissues moist during the healing period. Many manufactured nasal packs are large enough or in tight enough spaces to stay put on their own; others are secured outside the nose with thin strings taped to the outside of the nose.

Middle meatal spacers

Non-absorbable material inserted in the space between the middle turbinate and the side of the nasal cavity to help prevent collapse of the middle turbinate.

With the improvements in sinus surgery techniques, many surgeons do not use any nasal packing at all.

When nasal packing is placed in certain areas with non-adherent coverings, it can help reduce scar tissue formation in the nose. Small packings may be used to help hold open the space between the middle turbinate and the side of the nose; these are also called **middle meatal spacers**. Small packs typically are not noticed by patients, but large amounts of nasal packing can be quite uncomfortable. With the improvements in sinus surgery techniques, many surgeons do not use any nasal packing at all.

Nasal packing may be removed as early as 1 day after surgery or up to 7 days after surgery. While uncomfortable, packing removal is brief. Recently, packing materials that are absorbed or dissolve with nasal irrigations have been developed, which sometimes takes away the need for packing even in patients who need middle meatal spacers. Some commonly used packing materials are shown in **Figure 23**.

66: How do I prevent nosebleeds after surgery? What if my nose bleeds after sinus surgery?

After sinus surgery, do not blow your nose. Sneeze with your mouth open. This helps prevent pressure build-up in the nasal cavity. It also keeps air from being forced through the thin bony wall of the eye socket into the

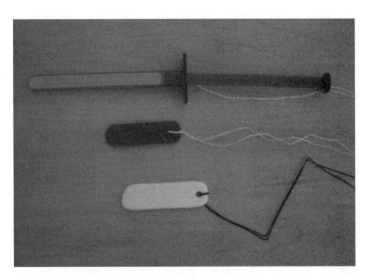

Figure 23 Samples of different nasal packing materials

skin under the eyes and into the skin around the eye, causing it to puff up and perhaps even feel "crunchy." Avoid strenuous activity or doing anything that will increase pressure in your head for about 2 weeks after surgery. Do not take aspirin, ibuprofen, or naproxen after surgery because they will reduce your ability to clot blood. Do not pick your nose and avoid inserting objects inside the nose. Crusts can be removed by nasal irrigation and dryness relieved with either the nasal irrigation or the use of a nasal saline spray.

Most nosebleeds stop on their own. If necessary, apply pressure to the two sides of the soft part of your nose and put your head down forward so that you avoid swallowing the blood, which will cause nausea. If it does not stop after 20 minutes, you should seek medical attention from your physician's office or a hospital emergency department.

67: What if I have changes in my vision after sinus surgery?

If you notice blurriness or double vision while in the recovery room, immediately notify the recovery room nurses or the surgeon so that they can evaluate you further. Blurriness or double vision may indicate an eye injury that requires prompt treatment. If you notice it after you get home, contact your surgeon immediately to discuss the symptoms. If he or she is not available, go to the nearest emergency department for evaluation.

Blurriness or double vision may indicate an eye injury that requires prompt treatment.

Direct injury to the globe of the eye or to the optic nerve is extremely rare. Changes in vision can vary from mild corneal abrasion on the surface of the eye, which can cause blurry vision, to injury to the muscles in the eye socket that move the eye, causing double vision. Bleeding within the eye socket during or after the surgery is a special concern; increased pressure within the eye will reduce blood flow to the optic nerve, which can result in blindness. Prompt identification of vision changes will hopefully reduce the long-term impact of the injury on your ability to see.

The type of treatment will depend on the cause of vision changes. Your physician may consult an ophthalmologist or request a CT scan. Corneal abrasions are usually treated with artificial tears and will generally heal on their own. Bleeding within the orbit (eye socket) requires immediate action to decrease the pressure within the eye. This may involve cutting the outer corner of the eye (lateral canthotomy) and operative reexploration to stop the bleeding and decompress the eye socket by removing some bone to help release pressure on the eye and the optic nerve. Injury to the muscles that move the eye is explored by the surgeon with an ophthalmologist and, if possible, the muscle is repaired. If the eye muscle injury cannot be repaired, then attempts to help "fuse" central gaze, which is when you are looking straight ahead, can be made using special glasses. Botulinum toxin or surgeries can also be performed to weaken the other eye muscles so that there is less opposing motion to pull the eye away from center.

68: What is empty nose syndrome?

Empty nose syndrome occurs when there has been extensive resection of the nasal cavity contents, including most, if not all, of the turbinates. The loss of the turbinate tissue leads to dryness of the nasal cavity because the surface area and volume of tissue available to warm and humidify the inhaled air is reduced. Crusts may develop within the nasal cavity as a result, which are uncomfortable and impede airflow through the nose.

...patients with empty nose syndrome paradoxically have a persistent sense of nasal obstruction.

Despite the large open empty nasal cavities, patients with empty nose syndrome paradoxically have a persistent sense of nasal obstruction. Normally, the turbinate tissues generate some resistance to air on inspiration, so the absence of the turbinates results in the loss of the sensation of air moving through the nasal cavities. Unfortunately, there is no way to reverse the anatomical changes caused by the removal of the turbinates. Management involves moisturizing and removing crusts in the nasal cavity with saline sprays or irrigations.

69. What is balloon sinuplasty?

Balloon sinuplasty

A form of sinus surgery in which small balloons are used to dilate sinus openings.

Fluoroscopy

The use of X-ray to produce an image on a monitor in real-time, rather than printing on film.

Balloon Sinuplasty, also called *catheter-based dilation of sinus ostia* or *functional endoscopic dilation of the sinuses,* is a new device that is guided into the sinuses with a special type of X-rays called **fluoroscopy** to dilate the sinus openings the same way angioplasty dilates the vessels on the heart. A hollow suction or positioning device is placed over the sinus opening using conventional nasal endoscopy in the operating room. Then, a guide wire is passed through the positioning device and into the sinus while watching the position of the guide wire on fluoroscopy. A small balloon catheter, shown in **Figure 24**, is passed over the guide wire that was placed in the sinus, also using fluoroscopy to confirm its location within the sinus. Then the balloon is slowly inflated so that it gradually dilates the opening to the sinus; the image of the balloon being inflated on a fluoroscopy screen is shown in **Figure 25**. The sinus can then be drained and the interior of the sinus examined using a nasal endoscope.

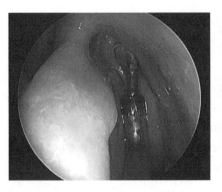

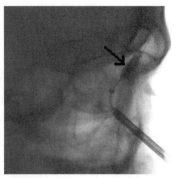

Figure 24 Balloon Sinuplasty™ catheter

Figure 25 X-ray image of balloon inflated inside the sinus openings

Balloon Sinuplasty involves little to no tissue removal inside the nose and sinuses. At the present time, it is used to open the frontal, maxillary, and sphenoid sinuses. It is not used for treating ethmoid sinus disease; in some cases, ethmoid sinus disease can be treated with conventional sinus surgery and the remainder of the sinuses treated with Balloon Sinuplasty. Because the technique was recently introduced, surgeons are still learning which patients it will work best for and when it is the appropriate choice of device for surgery. Situations for which Balloon Sinuplasty is usually not appropriate are cases of large nasal polyps or significant scarring from previous sinus surgery.

Long-term success rates are not yet available. However, studies conducted so far appear promising with many selected patients reporting good results. Patients who undergo Balloon Sinuplasty appear to have a little less pain and bleeding during the postoperative period. There are many new studies in progress that may soon help physicians better determine how the Balloon Sinuplasty device fits into the sinusitis management spectrum.

70. Will I have pain after sinus surgery?

Most patients feel some nasal stuffiness or pressure in the sinuses, but there should not be excruciating pain. The discomfort will usually improve after the first day or two. Pain medications will usually be provided for the postoperative period and should relieve most of the pain. If the pain cannot be controlled with pain medications, you should notify your physician as soon as possible.

Muffie's comments:

I took pain killers anticipating pain; I did not like the side effects so I stopped taking them. I only took three pills total. Then I switched to Tylenol for a few days. The pain did not restrict me in any way!

71. When should I expect to notice improvement? What is the post-operative care after sinus surgery?

Many patients feel improvement as early as immediately after surgery...

Many patients feel improvement as early as immediately after surgery, especially if a number of nasal polyps were removed to clear the nasal passage or if a large amount of mucus or pus was drained from the sinuses, which relieves sensation of pressure or pain in the face or head. However, surgery is only the beginning of the path to recovery for recalcitrant sinusitis, because the healing process will continue for months afterward. It can take several weeks for the swelling inside to subside. The sense of smell can take months to recover.

Most otolaryngologists will instruct you to begin nasal saline irrigations the day after surgery. Depending on the type of sinus problems you have, they may also prescribe antibiotics and/or steroids after surgery. Some physicians will also recommend the use of oral or topical nasal decongestants to help with the feeling of congestion in the nose that results from the mucosal swelling.

Diligent postoperative examination and sinus "debridements," or removal of debris inside the nose, will help maintain the sinus openings and prevent scar tissue formation. Most surgeons will see you during the first week after sinus surgery. During the first postoperative visit, if there is nasal packing, it will be removed. Nasal endoscopy will be performed and crusts, old blood, and old mucus present in the nose or sinus cavities will be suctioned out. Any developing scar tissue or small polyps will also be removed. Stents, which are tubes of material such as silicone or rubber used to help keep sinus drainage pathways open, are usually left in place for several weeks.

Diligent postoperative examination and sinus "debridements," or removal of debris inside the nose, will help maintain the sinus openings and prevent scar tissue formation.

Because the debridement can be uncomfortable even in the presence of topical anesthetics, it may be best to have someone drive you to the visit so that if you need to take pain medications before or after the procedure you will be able to do so without worrying that it will impair your ability to drive. The frequency of visits after the first visit will vary according to the condition of your nose and sinuses and how well the healing process is going. If you have a tendency to form a lot of scar tissue or if polyps redevelop quickly, you will require more frequent postoperative maintenance than someone who does not have these tendencies.

Muffie's comments:

Having had my second FESS, I learned that after care is THE most important step. Be diligent, and it will pay off!

72. When are "open" approaches to sinus surgery needed?

With certain anatomical variations of the sinuses, it may not be possible to completely perform sinus surgery from within the nose. For instance, if there is an extra sinus "cell" inside the frontal sinus that is further off to the side than usual, it might not be reached through standard endoscopic techniques. In addition, if sinusitis or sinusitis-like symptoms are caused by a tumor, either benign (not cancerous) or malignant (cancerous), an open approach may be needed. In cases of malignancy, an open approach facilitates complete removal of the cancer. Even with benign tumors, sometimes an external approach is needed to help with surgical access or visualization, though most of the procedure is being done with endoscopy. Fractures of the sinuses requiring repair are also fixed through open approaches.

Possible locations for incisions are inside the upper lip, along the side of the nose near the eye, above the eyebrow, or behind the hairline. Incisions to increase access or visualization of the frontal sinuses are usually small and located above the eyebrow. If there is a frontal sinus cancer or fracture, a long incision behind the front hairline is used. The external approach to the ethmoid sinuses is with an incision along the nose close to the eye. The incision inside the upper lip is used to get additional access to the maxillary sinus.

External approaches will almost always result in a visible scar. Recovery after procedures done after an external approach also often takes longer, and there will probably be more pain and possibly bleeding compared to endoscopic procedures. Numbness of the skin overlying the incision site is possible. In the approach to the maxillary

With certain anatomical variations of the sinuses, it may not be possible to completely perform sinus surgery from within the nose.

sinus, if the nerve supplying sensation to the upper lip and face is injured, those areas can be permanently numb. With the open procedure to the frontal sinus, there is a higher risk of CSF leak and double vision.

PART SIX

Living with and Preventing Sinusitis

How can I keep sinusitis from coming back?

Will I have to stay on medications
for sinusitis forever?

How do I optimize the condition
of my home to help improve my allergies?

More . . .

73: How can I keep sinusitis from coming back?

There are many ways to prevent sinusitis from coming back. Aggressive management of nasal mucosal inflammation is the most important. If you or someone in your household smokes, you or they should stop because substances in the smoke damage the cilia lining of the nose. Damaged cilia do not move well; mucus and bacteria can accumulate in the nose and sinuses, which can lead to sinusitis. Identify and control exposure to allergens as much as possible.

You should also avoid things that dry out the lining of the nose, such as dry indoor heat and medications that dehydrate you, such as diuretics. Stay hydrated by drinking plenty of fluids. Avoid things that cause the nasal mucosa to swell, such as allergens and alcohol.

Take all medications that your physician prescribes for you to prevent sinusitis, such as nasal steroids. If you have allergic rhinitis, asthma, cystic fibrosis, or any other diseases related to sinusitis, maintain good control over those conditions. Try to avoid sick people if possible and wash hands frequently if it is unavoidable. Follow up with your physician as scheduled so that he or she can help you prevent problems from developing.

74: Will I have to stay on medications for sinusitis forever?

Inflammation represents a significant component of sinusitis. Medications that help with inflammation may be required long term to help reduce inflammation in the nasal cavities to make sinusitis less likely to occur.

Because there is presently no way to permanently change the lining of the nose and sinuses with medications, medications must be taken continuously to maintain the anti-inflammatory effects.

75: How do I optimize the condition of my home to help improve my allergies?

Although you can't do anything to limit your exposure to outdoor allergens, you can improve the condition of the air inside your home with air conditioners and air purifiers. All carpets should be vacuumed at least once a week and more often, if possible. Room curtains need to be cleaned and linens washed frequently. High-efficiency particulate air filters used in air purifiers may help clean the air in your home if you have environmental allergens. Limit or remove indoor plants and keep dander-producing animals out of your home. Change woolen bed linens and pillows with feathers to ones made of cotton or synthetic fibers. Use special plastic mattress and pillow covers if you have a dust mite allergy.

Viruses, bacteria, mold, and fungi are present nearly everywhere and can survive in nearly every climate, so it is difficult to avoid them. Bathrooms, kitchens, and basements are where bacteria and fungi are most likely to grow in the home, so it is important to keep those areas clean. In the kitchens, keep garbage cans, the spaces under the sink and the refrigerator, and cutting boards as clean and dry as possible. Make sure that you use a clean sponge or cloth to avoid spreading bacteria or mold when wiping your hands, your silverware, pots and pans, dinnerware, and cooking utensils. In the bathrooms, keep tub and sink surfaces, bathroom rugs, and shower curtains free of mold and bacteria. Avoid carpeting in the

Viruses, bacteria, mold, and fungi are present nearly everywhere and can survive in nearly every climate, so it is difficult to avoid them.

basement because the padding or the carpet itself is susceptible to mold formation. Keep the surfaces of the washer and dryer from accumulating moisture if possible.

76: How is allergy testing done, and how does it help sinusitis? What is allergy immunotherapy?

If your symptoms suggest allergic disease or you notice that there are certain types of things such as molds or pollens that irritate the lining of your nose, your physician will send you for allergy testing. Allergy testing will help determine what substances you have a reaction to and help guide treatment. Knowing what your allergens are will help you avoid them. Continued exposure to allergens and persistent allergy symptoms will cause sinusitis and asthma symptoms to worsen.

Knowing what your allergens are will help you avoid them.

Allergy testing may be done in either an allergist's or an otolaryngolgist's office. It can be categorized into two methods. The first type is done by drawing blood and sending it to a lab to be tested; this is called a **radioallergosorbent test (RAST)**. It measures the amount of an antibody that your body makes to fight allergens. The second method involves using small needles or a small batch of needles to make skin pricks or injections of different things to which you may have an allergic reaction. Identifying allergens and undergoing allergy immunotherapy or using allergy medications helps reduce intranasal inflammation and thus your susceptibility to sinusitis.

Radioallergosorbent test (RAST)

Blood test that measures the amount of an antibody that your body makes to fight a particular allergen to determine if you are allergic to it.

If exposure to allergens is unavoidable and cannot be controlled with medications such as nasal steroids or antihistamines, allergy immunotherapy to desensitize you to the allergens may be necessary. **Allergy immunotherapy** involves a series of injections of a custom-made solution of antigens to which you are allergic. The dose that you are treated with is very small initially and usually administered twice a week. Over time, as you become less sensitive to the antigens, your physician will increase the amounts of the antigen, make the solution more concentrated, and decrease the frequency of the shots. The length of time to completing desensitization can be as long as 2 years.

The most serious risk is an anaphylactic allergic reaction, which causes swelling in your breathing passageways. For that reason, allergy shots are usually given under doctor's supervision, usually by a nurse. The medical office where the allergy immunotherapy is done should have all necessary equipment and medications, in case of a life-threatening anaphylactic allergic response.

77: What should I do if I need to fly with sinusitis?

Air travel causes pressure changes in the sinuses and the ear. These changes need to be equalized by air passing into or out of the sinuses and the Eustachian tubes, which connect to the ear. Equalizing pressure may be more difficult when flying with a sinus infection if the sinuses are closed off. The inflammation from sinusitis also can cause the Eustachian tubes to be unable to function properly, causing ear pain.

Pain or pressure in the sinuses is typically the worst during descent, when cabin pressure increases and air needs to enter the blocked sinus openings. You should avoid flying with sinusitis if possible. The infection may

Allergy immunotherapy

A progressive series of injections containing increasing amounts of a substance to which the doctor is attempting to desensitize the patient.

Allergy immunotherapy involves a series of injections of a custom-made solution of antigens to which you are allergic.

You should avoid flying with sinusitis if possible.

be exacerbated by the air conditions on the plane; if you do not have an infection, but are prone to them, then flying can precipitate an infection.

If you must fly, you can try oral decongestants 30 minutes before the flight and nasal saline sprays during the flight to make it less uncomfortable. Using a nasal decongestant spray such as oxymetazoline (Afrin) before take-off may help. Chewing on gum or swallowing will help open the Eustachian tubes. Rinsing the nose with saline after the flight will also help because the air inside the passenger cabin is typically dry and recirculated. These measures may be useful for preventing sinus infections if you are prone to them, even if you are not sick at the time of the flight. If you have frequent episodes of sinusitis, a short course of oral steroids may be beneficial, starting a few days before the flight.

Paula's comments:

When flying, I spray my nose with Afrin and take Sudafed. I also chew gum.

78: Can I scuba dive or swim if I have sinus problems?

Scuba diving can present a problem for sinusitis patients due to difficulty with the pressure changes in the sinuses.

Chlorine in pools can irritate the nasal passageways. Furthermore, both chlorinated and fresh water may contain microorganisms and pollutants that will irritate the nasal mucosa and can cause infection. After you swim, your nose should be irrigated with saline to cleanse it and prevent inflammation and infection.

Scuba diving can present a problem for sinusitis patients due to difficulty with the pressure changes in the sinuses. Patients with nasal congestion, sinusitis, or allergies often cannot pressurize the ears and sinuses properly. This results in either "sinus squeeze," which is facial pain, or "ear squeeze," which is ear pain. If a "squeeze" occurs, it is important to ascend enough to relieve the pressure or permanent damage to the ears or sinuses could occur. You should avoid diving during a cold, sinusitis, or acute worsening of allergies.

Tina's comments:

Although I probably had chronic sinusitis most of my life, I grew up in a swimming pool. My nose was always more stuffy after a swim practice, and I always attributed it to the chlorine. However, it never impacted my swim schedule.

I am also an avid free diver, which is similar to scuba diving except that no air supply is used. When free diving, I quickly descend and ascend, causing rapid changes in air pressure. Sometimes I can feel needle-like pain in my right cheek and still be able to continue with my descent only to hear a popping sound. Once back on the surface, I realize I have a bloody nose. Most recently while free diving in Kauai, my frontal sinuses could not equalize and I felt excruciating pain in the middle of my forehead. The pain was so severe that I could not go any deeper but instead could only hover around 20 feet. Sometimes nasal decongestants help. Get your sinuses used to the pressure by slowly advancing downward a little at a time. In general, sinus squeeze can be very frustrating.

79: How do I ease sinus symptoms if I can't see a doctor right away?

Stay hydrated by drinking plenty of fluids. Steam inhalation may help loosen secretions and ease nasal congestion. Avoid blowing your nose hard because that will simply cause the lining to swell more. Stop smoking and avoid people who are smoking.

Over-the-counter oral and topical decongestants may help alleviate the symptoms by decreasing nasal congestion. Nasal saline irrigations will help decrease nasal congestion and wash away thick mucus. Guaifenesin will thin secretions and make them easier to clear. Be careful when you take over-the-counter cold or allergy preparations because many contain more than one medication and you can inadvertently overdose on one. Remember that nasal decongestants should be used for only 3 to 5 days; if used longer, they can cause rebound congestion.

80: What if my ears bother me when I get sinusitis?

The Eustachian tubes, which equalize the pressure in the ears and which connect the ear to the nose, may not function properly when you have sinusitis.

The Eustachian tubes, which equalize the pressure in the ears and which connect the ear to the nose, may not function properly when you have sinusitis. This causes the ears to either feel stopped up or to "pop" inappropriately when the lining of the nose is inflamed. Eustachian tube problems often respond to the use of oral or nasal decongestants.

The other possibility is that an ear infection has developed in the ears at the same time as the sinuses or if there are polyps, that the polyps are blocking the Eustachian tube. You should be examined by a physician to determine what is causing the ear pain because the ear infection may require antibiotics and polyps will probably require a treatment with steroids.

81: What if my nasal polyps come back?

Unfortunately, nasal polyps often recur.

Unfortunately, nasal polyps often recur. Important therapies that may help prevent recurrence are allergy treatment if you have allergies. For patients with aspirin-sensitive asthma, aspirin desensitization slows recurrence. Topical steroids, the allergy medication montelukast (Singulair) and the macrolide antibiotics clarithromycin (Biaxin) and azithromycin (Zithromax) are medications that have been shown to help prevent polyp recurrence.

If polyps are small and in an easily accessed position inside the nose, the otolaryngologist may be able to simply remove them with a nasal endoscope and a small pair of forceps during the office visit. Oral steroids may be prescribed if there are larger polyps. Nasal steroid washes, which are being used by some allergists and otolaryngolgists, also seem to help reduce polyp size and prevent regrowth. If the polyps are very large, the only way to relieve symptoms such as nasal obstruction may be to perform sinus surgery.

82: What if I keep getting sinusitis after my sinus surgery?

Sinusitis is a disease affecting the lining of the nose. Surgery addresses anatomical issues that may predispose you to infection and may secondarily improve the condition of the lining of your nose. However, because the lining of your nose is the same after surgery, it may still react the same way to environmental insults such as bacteria, dust, and irritants. Because most people catch a few viral colds each year (which are hard to prevent), those colds may precipitate a sinus infection. Hopefully, with open sinus drainage pathways, the sinus infections will be less severe.

Evaluation for immune system diseases should be considered in people with recurrent severe infections because sometimes people are prone to recurrent respiratory tract

Evaluation for immune system diseases should be considered in people with recurrent severe infections...

infections due to immunodeficiencies. Some immuno-deficiency diseases can be quite subtle and will require substantial effort to uncover. There are medications and treatments that can help people diagnosed with these conditions to strengthen their immune systems.

Efforts should be made to comply with a regimen of nasal rinses, allergy medications (if appropriate), and frequent hand washing to minimize the chance of recurrence. Instituting measures to control environmental contributors to allergy symptoms will reap significant benefits. If symptoms keep returning, your otolaryngologist may send you to a rhinologist, someone who focuses his or her practice exclusively on the management of nasal and sinus disease.

Paula's comments:

My asthma is triggered when I have a sinus infection and vice versa. I increase my inhaler use and my nasal rinses.

I feel we need to understand that chronic sinusitis is difficult to live with. We need to do our best to continue our regular lifestyle and get plenty of exercise. A positive attitude helps.

83: Does the food I eat affect sinusitis? What about alcohol?

Identifying food allergies is often difficult because the symptoms are often mild. Milk and wheat allergies can lead to excess mucus production and postnasal drip. The excess mucus can block sinus drainage, which leads to infection.

Definitively demonstrating food allergies is hard to do; skin testing and RAST blood testing have both been used with variable success. A trial of an elimination diet for 2–4 weeks is often necessary. All foods containing the suspected offender should be eliminated from the diet. This can be difficult because there are preservatives in most prepared foods; careful reading of the ingredient labels will help. You should notice a substantial improvement in your symptoms if food allergies are the underlying cause.

Patients with chronic rhinitis or chronic sinusitis often notice that their symptoms worsen when they drink red wine or the darker types of alcohol. The main problem noticed is an increase in nasal stuffiness. This is believed to be caused by the dilation of inflamed blood vessels in the nose. It also could be an allergic response. Either way, it is probably best to avoid red wine and alcohol to prevent additional nasal congestion when you have sinusitis.

Muffie's comment:

That is why I stick to white wine!

84: Can heartburn or reflux cause sinusitis?

The medical term for heartburn is **gastroesophageal reflux disease (GERD)**. Reflux occurs when the acidic contents of the stomach travel back up into the esophagus. When the acid travels high enough to affect the voice box and throat, it is called **laryngopharyngeal reflux (LPR)**. LPR can cause hoarseness, frequent throat clearing, the sensation of a lump in the throat, and a cough. It can cause the sensation of a postnasal drip, which causes it to be mistaken for sinusitis.

Patients with chronic rhinitis or chronic sinusitis often notice that their symptoms worsen when they drink red wine or the darker types of alcohol.

Gastroesophageal reflux disease (GERD)

Occurs when gastric acid and enzymes from the stomach back up inside the esophagus.

Treatment for LPR includes both lifestyle and dietary changes. These include not lying down for several hours after eating, sleeping with the head of the bed elevated, and eating smaller meals more frequently. Alcohol and caffeine consumption should be reduced, as well as tomato and citrus products. Alcohol can further relax the esophageal sphincter. Tomato and citrus products are very acidic. Treatment may also include the use of medications to reduce acid production or to neutralize acids.

85: What are some of the latest trends in research for sinusitis?

An exciting recent development in research on sinusitis suggests that biofilms may play a role on sinusitis. **Biofilms** are made of groups of bacteria that form a protective and adherent matrix. They are difficult for antibiotics to penetrate. Plaque is one example that most people have at some point. These biofilms have been demonstrated in many types of infection, including chronic sinusitis. Understanding the role of biofilms and how to better disperse them may improve the effectiveness of chronic sinusitis treatment.

Robotically assisted surgery being increasingly used in heart and prostate procedures has reduced recovery times for the patients. Using robotic arms to perform the surgery gives the surgeon, who sits in a virtual reality booth to operate the instruments, finer control of small instruments. In time, the instruments may become small enough to fit inside the nose and have sufficient range of motion to allow work inside the nose.

Further enhancements in image-guided surgery with real-time imaging are in the pipeline. Intraoperative MRI is now available and can be used during surgery to get an image of the sinus tissues being operated on. CT scanners also are being developed that are small enough to fit in the operating room and can rotate around the head to take an intraoperative image. These intraoperative scans can show the surgeons the progress they have made. The scans can then be loaded into an image-guidance system or be merged into existing scans on the image-guidance system.

Topical medications for the possible regeneration of the linings of the nose are being explored in animal models. The hope is that use of these medications will be able to restore the presence of normal and functional mucosal lining within the sinuses damaged by surgery. With the restoration of normal mucosa, normal mucociliary clearance can resume.

Novel delivery devices for nasal medications to ensure a wider, more uniform distribution have been developed. Nebulizers are already available commercially, and studies are underway to determine if their use confers any advantage. Technology is also being used to develop spray bottle medication delivery devices that coat the nasal cavity more effectively; these devices are undergoing testing and will soon be available for clinical use.

An allergy vaccine for an allergen that causes hay fever is currently in the early stages of large-scale clinical trials testing and is showing promising results. There are also genetic studies as well as studies examining the possible chemicals contributing to the development of sinusitis that may impact how sinusitis is treated in the future.

PART SEVEN

Complementary and Alternative Therapies

Do vitamins prevent sinusitis?

Can acupuncture or acupressure be used to treat sinusitis?

Are there herbal therapies for sinusitis?

More . . .

86: Do vitamins prevent sinusitis?

Multivitamins have been shown in two small pediatric studies to have a positive impact on chronic sinusitis when used in combination with cod liver oil. Vitamin C by itself is believed to shorten the duration and reduce the severity of a cold. However, no objective studies have demonstrated this claim.

... vitamins are pharmacologically active and can interact with other medications.

Zinc is also thought to help prevent infections. It is available in both oral and topical forms. Studies seem to indicate that the duration of a cold is shortened if a zinc nasal spray is used within 24 hours of onset; the disadvantage is that the spray must be used frequently, every 4 hours. There are a few studies that link the use of zinc nasal sprays to the increased risk of the loss of the sense of smell, though the loss could also be attributed to the presence of respiratory infection. Zinc sprays should be used in accordance with the instructions and stopped immediately if any changes in the sense of smell are noticed.

Acupuncture

A technique based on restoring the balance of the body's life force by stimulating specific points with needles.

Though vitamins are sold without a prescription and are generally safe, vitamins are pharmacologically active and can interact with other medications. You should check with your physician and your pharmacist if you are taking them at the same time as other medications. Also, if you are planning to have surgery, you should stop taking vitamin E before surgery in order to prevent excessive bleeding.

Acupuncture is a technique based on restoring the balance of ch'i, a life force that flows along meridians on the body and is disrupted by illness.

87: Can acupuncture or acupressure be used to treat sinusitis?

Acupuncture is a technique based on restoring the balance of ch'i, a life force that flows along meridians on the body and is disrupted by illness. This is achieved by the insertion of long, thin needles into surface points on the meridians that are connections to organs to stimulate them. Although no one knows how acupuncture works, there are several theories. One commonly held theory is that it causes the release of **endorphins**, which are naturally occurring chemicals that bind the same areas as narcotics, thereby relieving pain. Anecdotally, there are indications that acupuncture may help relieve pressure and pain caused by sinusitis; however, there are not any good studies supporting the use of acupuncture for the treatment of sinusitis.

A survey of acupuncture practitioners indicated that it is a common indication for acupuncture and those surveyed indicated that the patients had good responses to therapy. One small study comparing acupuncture to conventional sinusitis medication therapy showed a slight advantage to conventional therapy for treatment of symptoms. There was also a significant difference noted on the objective measure, which was examining the amount of swelling in the sinus linings by CT scan.

Endorphins

Naturally occurring chemicals that bind the same areas as narcotics, thereby relieving pain.

Acupressure is similar to acupuncture and is based on the same principles. However, instead of needles, pressure is applied to the appropriate points for a specified period of time. An advantage of acupressure over acupuncture is that the patient can be taught to perform acupressure on the points for him or herself.

Acupressure

Technique based on restoring the balance of the body's life force by stimulating specific points with pressure.

Paula's comments:

I had acupuncture for 3 years. It did not cure my sinusitis, but it helped to relieve some of my symptoms, such as pressure in my head and a stuffy nose. I felt good after each treatment.

88: Are there herbal therapies for sinusitis?

Several herbal medications may be used in the management of sinusitis.

Several herbal medications may be used in the management of sinusitis. Bromelain is a compound from pineapples that is thought to reduce inflammation. Several studies done in the 1960s showed that patients had greater sinusitis symptom relief when taking bromelain in addition to antibiotics than when taking antibiotics alone. A more recent pediatric study demonstrated similar results.

Echinacea is a purple coneflower that grows from a black root in North America. It is thought to improve the immune system and prevent infections from developing. Echinacea is used for the treatment of colds and allergies, sometimes in combination with goldenseal or vitamin C.

Goldenseal is a perennial North American plant with golden roots that is also used for the treatment of cold and flu. It is believed to have antibacterial and anti-inflammatory properties. Its active ingredients are hydrastine and berberine. The medical use of goldenseal originated with the Cherokee group of Native Americans, who used it as a wash for skin infections and wounds. It is often used in preparations for genitourinary and gastrointestinal problems.

Use caution if using herbal supplements because the Food and Drug Administration regulation of herbal supplements is limited.

Use caution if using herbal supplements because the Food and Drug Administration regulation of herbal supplements is limited. Ingredients and purity will sometimes vary. If you do use a supplement, you should notify your physician because the herbs are pharmacologically active and can interact with other medications that you take. Furthermore, if you are planning surgery, you should be aware that ginger, garlic, gingko, and ginseng are known to increase bleeding. These herbs should be stopped about 2 weeks prior to surgery. You should also check any herbal preparations carefully for the presence of aspirin because many may use it as a component; if there is aspirin, it should be stopped at least a week before surgery.

89: Can stress relief techniques help sinusitis?

Emotional and physical stress tend to lead to exacerbations of chronic illnesses such as chronic sinusitis. There are many methods that can help reduce stress. Examples include yoga, tai chi, meditation, and biofeedback. Regular exercise such as running or biking may also relieve stress. Each individual should experiment with the different methods to try to find something that is effective in reducing stress and that you can do consistently.

Emotional and physical stress tend to lead to exacerbations of chronic illnesses such as chronic sinusitis.

90: Could aromatherapy help my sinus symptoms? Can steam therapy help?

Aromatherapy is the use of highly concentrated and pure extracts that are either heated as oils, burned as candles, or added to hot water. Moist, warm air is generated and may relieve sinus congestion and moisten the lining of the nose, loosening secretions. Oils such as menthol and eucalyptus in particular may also help relieve congestion.

Inhaling steam loosens mucus that accumulates within the breathing passageways. Steam machines for the face are available commercially, but one could also boil a pot of water and then breathe in the steam for a few minutes after turning it off; draping a towel over the head while doing this may help. Do not put your face directly

Inhaling steam loosens mucus that accumulates within the breathing passageways.

over boiling water because the steam may be hot enough to burn you. An alternative is a long, hot shower, which will have a similarly beneficial effect.

91: What is myofascial release therapy?

Myofascial release is a manual massage technique. The concept is that the bonds between the fascia, integument, muscles, and bones are stretched and released, for the purpose of eliminating pain, increasing range of motion, and balancing the body. **Fascia** is composed of connective tissue that covers and connects the different muscles, organs, and tissue structures in the body.

Restrictions in the fascia are caused by injuries, stress, inflammation, trauma, and poor posture. Because the fascia is an interconnected web, the restriction or tightness to fascia at a particular place can spread over time to other places in the body. The goal of myofascial release is to release fascia restriction and restore its tissue health.

92: What are xylitol and capsaicin, and how do they help sinusitis?

Xylitol, also called wood or birch sugar, is a sugar alcohol that has antibacterial properties. Xylitol is extracted from corn husks, berries, birch trees, and plums. It is most commonly used as a sugar substitute in gum and candy and is also used in oral dental products, because it has been shown to have a beneficial effect on dental caries.

Xylitol has been sold in nasal spray forms and is believed to help reduce bacteria within the nasal cavities by making it difficult for bacteria to adhere to the mucosal linings. One animal study, using rabbits, has shown that the presence of xylitol seems to enhance bacterial killing. Of note, it can have a laxative effect when taken in large oral doses.

Capsaicin is a chemical found in hot and spicy foods including hot peppers such as jalapeño peppers. Due its effect on the nose, which includes inducing rhinorrhea and reducing nasal congestion, over-the-counter topical sprays, and oral supplements have been developed for the treatment of sinusitis. Some studies showed that it has an effect on a chemical that is part of the pain pathway. However, no major benefits have been found in objective studies on capsaicin.

COMPLEMENTARY AND ALTERNATIVE THERAPIES

Capsaicin

Chemical component of plants present in hot peppers that can be an irritant to skin and mucosa, but may also have topical analgesic properties.

PART EIGHT

Special Situations

How is treating sinusitis in children different from treating an adult?

What is cystic fibrosis, and how is sinusitis different in cystic fibrosis?

How is sinusitis different in the elderly?

More...

93: How is treating sinusitis in children different from treating an adult?

As in adults, the sinus drainage pathways in children can be blocked and lead to sinusitis. The most common causes of sinusitis are colds and other viral infections. Diagnosing sinusitis may be more challenging in children because most children only have nasal discharge. Physicians usually prefer to treat suspected infection rather than perform radiologic studies to confirm the diagnosis.

The same medications used in adults may be adjusted in dose for children.

The same medications used in adults may be adjusted in dose for children. The antibiotic exceptions are the tetracyclines and quinolones. Tetracycline can cause permanent discoloration of the teeth in children under 8 years of age, and quinolones can cause damage to joints and to cartilage development. Topical nasal steroid sprays can be used safely in children over the age of 2 and do not appear to have any impact on long-term growth.

Adenoids

Hump of lymphoid tissue in the back of the nose.

The **adenoids** are a hump of tissue in the back of the nose that is the same as the tissue that grows in the tonsils. The adenoids can sometimes become large enough to block nasal breathing and cause snoring, nasal drainage, and even sinusitis by harboring bacteria. Repeated infections can occur if the adenoids remain enlarged and act as a reservoir for bacteria. **Adenoidectomy**, a short outpatient procedure, is the removal of this tissue through the mouth.

Adenoidectomy

Removal of enlarged lymphoid tissue present in the back of the nose.

Sinus surgery is performed less often in children but has also been shown to be successful. Sinus surgery is different in children because the frontal and sphenoid sinuses may not be fully formed and the ethmoid and maxillary sinuses are much smaller and higher in location than they are in adults. Also, initially, there were concerns that altering the bony structures of the sinuses would negatively impact facial growth; however, there are studies showing that was not true.

CF is a genetic disorder that presents itself in childhood and frequently causes nasal polyps. Children with nasal polyps need to be tested for CF. This is done by a sweat chloride test, which tests the amount of salt in their perspiration.

94: What is cystic fibrosis, and how is sinusitis different in cystic fibrosis?

Cystic fibrosis (CF) is a recessive inherited disorder that causes abnormalities in secretions produced by the lungs, pancreas, liver, and reproductive tract. Very thick mucus is produced by the nose and the lungs, which clogs the breathing passageways and leads to repeated infections such as pneumonia and sinusitis. CF patients usually have onset of rhinosinusitis sometime in childhood, but there are some people with milder versions of CF that do not have problems until adulthood. Therefore, young adults with serious sinus disease should also be screened for CF with a genetic blood test.

Cystic fibrosis (CF)

Recessive inherited disorder causing abnormalities in the lungs, sinuses, pancreas, liver, and reproductive tract.

Many CF patients have nasal polyps. The polyps usually recur after surgery and can be very difficult to control. More antibiotic-resistant infections are common in patients with CF because of the many antibiotic courses they receive over their lifetime. Because CF patients are more prone to pneumonia than most patients, sinusitis also can lead to an episode of pneumonia due to the infected mucus draining into the lungs. CF patients may benefit from using nebulized antibiotics that send topical antibiotics not only into the nose, but also the lungs. Frequent nasal irrigations may help thin nasal secretions and clear them out of the nasal cavity.

CF patients are more likely to require prolonged courses of antibiotics and possibly even require the placement of a long-term intravenous catheter. Functional endoscopic sinus surgery is usually of benefit when the symptoms become severe. The need for revision surgery is almost a certainty in most patients. Maximizing control over sinusitis is especially important in patients with CF to minimize the risk of additional damage to the lungs.

Maximizing control over sinusitis is especially important in patients with CF to minimize the risk of additional damage to the lungs.

95: How is sinusitis different in the elderly?

The nose undergoes changes as a person ages. Because the tip of the nose often droops in the elderly from weakening of the cartilages, this can narrow the space through which air can flow. The nose is often drier from atrophy of the nasal mucous glands. Fortunately, sensitivity to allergens diminishes as a person gets older. However, the elderly are as likely as younger adults to get sinus infections. If they are hospitalized frequently, they may be more likely to develop an infection from an antibiotic-resistant organism.

Sinusitis in the elderly is treated with the same medications as other adults. Because most elderly patients have more than one medical condition, it is imperative to check for medication interactions before starting any medication for sinusitis. It may also be necessary to adjust to a lower dose of an antibiotic to compensate for a slower metabolism. If medical treatments do not adequately improve the sinusitis, sinus surgery is still an option. Many elderly patients do well after sinus surgery if they had appropriate preoperative medical evaluation with diagnostic testing.

96: What about HIV infection and sinusitis?

HIV-positive patients have impaired mucociliary function, which means that they cannot effectively clear mucus and organisms from their sinuses. Approximately 80 percent of patients with acquired immune deficiency syndrome (AIDS) have chronic sinusitis. Sinusitis in AIDS patients is often difficult to manage, and sinus surgery is less likely to be successful at preventing future infections.

Infections are usually caused by similar organisms as in sinusitis patients without HIV. However, less-common infection-causing organisms such as cryptococcus, cytomegalovirus, and fungal species also are often found. Therefore, it is important to take cultures during an infection if possible. This allows selection of an antibiotic or antifungal medication that the organism is sensitive to and to determine if there are multiple simultaneous infections. Because sinusitis can spread quickly to adjacent tissues in patients who are immunocompromised and cause complications, it is treated aggressively. In particular, fungal sinusitis in a patient with immunosuppression can rapidly invade the eye and the brain and must be removed promptly.

Approximately 80 percent of patients with AIDS have chronic sinusitis.

97. What if I get sinusitis while I am pregnant?

Due to increased blood and fluid volume during pregnancy, women may notice an increase in nasal congestion. This can be treated with nasal saline sprays or irrigations. Patients with severe nasal congestion may also consider using certain nasal steroids. Because this increased nasal congestion can lead to obstruction of the sinus ostia, pregnant women with a history of sinusitis may notice an increase in their symptoms or the frequency of infection.

Though there is a general reluctance to prescribe medications to pregnant women, it is usually safe to give medications after the first trimester. There are several antibiotics and decongestants that appear to be safe for use during pregnancy. However, there are also some that are clearly contraindicated for use in pregnancy. It is important to consult your obstetrician prior to taking any medications.

98: How does my sinusitis affect my asthma?

Asthma is a chronic lung condition in which the lungs become intermittently inflamed and constricted in response to specific triggers. These triggers can include animals, pollens, pollution, dust, cold, or exercise. The cause of asthma is not known, but asthma seems to be increasing in prevalence in the population.

The symptoms of asthma are gasping and wheezing. The frequency and severity of asthma attacks can vary widely among those affected. In the milder cases, asthma can be treated with an albuterol inhaler on an as-needed basis to dilate the airways. At its worst, asthma may cause the patient to have episodes requiring intravenous steroids, airway intubation, and hospitalization. Many people with asthma also have sinusitis; about 75 percent of patients with asthma report sinusitis symptoms.

Asthma frequently worsens during or after colds or acute sinusitis. Treatment of sinusitis with medications often concurrently improves the asthma. Sinus surgery often has a beneficial effect for patients with asthma by improving the asthma symptoms and reducing the need for inhaled medications.

The aspirin triad, called "Samter's triad," consists of nasal polyps, aspirin allergy, and asthma. Nasal polyps tend to be much worse and have a higher recurrence rate than in patients who do not have this triad. People with this triad react to aspirin and related medications such as ibuprofen or naproxen with gastric upset, asthma, or allergic reactions. Selecting the appropriate therapy for the aspirin triad can be very complicated because more than one disease process is involved. Aspirin densensitization appears to be of benefit in delaying recurrence of nasal polyps.

The aspirin triad, called "Samter's triad," consists of nasal polyps, aspirin allergy, and asthma.

Tina's comments:

My asthma always worsens when I have a sinus infection. Often I can tell I am coming down with a sinus infection because my asthma flares and is more difficult to control.

Paula's comments:

I have adult-onset asthma, and it definitely contributes to my sinus infections. My asthma triggers when I'm having a sinus infection and vice versa. I increase my inhalers and my nasal rinses.

99: What is inverted papilloma, and how is it treated? What about sinus cancers?

Nasal and sinus tumors can initially appear with symptoms very similar to sinusitis. Inverted papilloma is the most common benign tumor of the sinuses and appears very similar to nasal polyps. Benign means that the tumor is not cancerous. However, inverted papilloma often grows rapidly, erodes the surrounding bone, and presses on the adjacent eye and brain. A small percentage of inverted papillomas may harbor a small cancer called **squamous cell carcinoma**; inverted papilloma can also transform into squamous cell carcinoma.

Squamous cell carcinoma

Form of cancer that arises from the cells on the skin or lining the surfaces of the gastrointestinal and respiratory tracts.

Treatment is complete removal of the inverted papilloma, which often can be achieved through endoscopic surgery. External incisions are rarely necessary. A small amount of normal tissue surrounding the inverted papilloma is usually removed because leaving just a few cells of the inverted papilloma can allow complete regrowth. With endoscopic resection, according to several studies, the recurrence rate hovers between 6–12 percent.

Cancers that arise from the nose and sinuses are rare.

Cancers that arise from the nose and sinuses are rare. Sinusitis may be present because of the blockage of the sinus drainage pathways by the tumor. Treatment is complete excision of the cancer. In some cases, this can be done endoscopically. In cases where the tumor is very large or involves the bone of the eye socket or skull base, it may have to be done either with external excisions or a combined external and endoscopic approach. Depending on the type of tumor, radiation treatment may follow surgery.

Arden's comments:

I had an initial procedure for removal of my inverted papilloma polyp and a follow-up procedure to remove the remaining affected tissue. After a follow-up surveillance examination, another suspect area was found. Tissue samples of this area were taken to determine if any inverted papilloma cells remain. If the biopsy is positive, additional affected tissue will need to be removed. I realize that I will need to be followed for several years because of the potential for recurrence of the inverted papilloma polyp.

100: What rare disorders may include sinusitis as part of the disease?

Wegener's granulomatosis is a rare disease that causes the formation of bead-like clumps of inflamed tissue called granulomas throughout the body. They form in the nose and sinuses, the lungs, and the kidneys. Granulomas form in the small and medium-sized blood vessels of the body and lead to the destruction of adjacent tissues. The linings of the nose are thinned, leading to frequent nosebleeds, the formation of crusts, and in the worst cases, destruction of the cartilaginous nasal septum, which leads to a depressed nasal bridge, which is called a **saddle nose**. Wegener's is confirmed with the c-ANCA blood test and/or nasal biopsy. Wegener's granulomatosis is treated with oral steroids and immunosuppressants.

Sarcoidosis is another rare granulomatous disease that causes beads of inflamed tissue to form throughout the body. Granulomas may occur in the nose and sinuses and contribute to the development of sinusitis. Most often, it is diagnosed from changes seen on a chest X-ray. The diagnosis is confirmed by testing angiotensin-converting enzyme levels in the blood. Sometimes sarcoidosis is identified from tissue removed during sinus surgery. Sarcoidosis is treated with oral steroids to reduce the inflammation.

Primary ciliary dyskinesia (Kartagener's syndrome) is a genetic disorder that causes a structural defect in the cilia, causing them to beat ineffectually. This leads to the accumulation of mucus, which then contributes to sinus infection and the formation of nasal polyps. Because cilia are also present in the lungs and the reproductive tract, patients with this disorder are prone to chronic cough and pneumonia and may have fertility problems.

Wegener's granulomatosis
A rare disease that causes clumps of inflamed tissue to form throughout the body.

Saddle nose
Depression of the nasal dorsum caused by destruction of the cartilage of the nasal septum.

Sarcoidosis
A rare disease that causes beads of inflamed tissue to form in the body.

Primary ciliary dyskinesia
Genetic disorder causing defective cilia to be unable to beat effectively.

Sinus infections are common in patients with Wegener's granulomatosis, sarcoidosis, and PCD; these infections are treated the same way as for other adult patients. Sinus surgery is indicated if the lesions from Wegener's or sarcoidosis become large enough to block the sinuses. Sinus surgery is also very effective for PCD, but recurrent disease is expected.

Useful
Web Sites

American Academy of Allergy,
Asthma & Immunology
555 East Wells Street, Suite 1100
Milwaukee, WI 53202-3823
1-800-822-ASMA (1-800-822-2762)
www.aaaai.org

This Web site has a directory of allergists and also has patient information.

American Academy of Family Physicians
P.O. Box 11210
Shawnee Mission, KS 66207-1210
1-800-274-2237
www.aafp.org

An older article (1998) published in the society journal that describes functional endoscopic sinus surgery: www.aafp.org/afp/980901ap/slack.html

An article published in the society journal on adult rhinosinusitis: www.aafp.org/afp/20010101/69.html

An article published in the society journal on allergic versus nonallergic rhinitis:
www.aafp.org/afp/20060501/1583.html

American Academy of Otolaryngology—
Head and Neck Surgery, Inc.
One Prince Street
Alexandria, VA 22314-3357
703-836-4444
www.entnet.org

The patient information section has numerous articles on sinusitis, sinus surgery, septoplasty, and inferior turbinate reduction; there are also diagrams explaining normal sinus anatomy. The "Find a Doctor" directory will help you find an otolaryngologist and will also show you the physician's credentials.

American College of Allergy, Asthma & Immunology

85 West Algonquin Road, Suite 550
Arlington Heights, IL 60005
847-427-1200
www.acaai.org/public

This is a large organization for allergists/immunologists.

American Rhinologic Society

9 Sunset Terrace
Warwick, NY 10990
845-988-1631
www.american-rhinologic.org/patientinfo.phtml

This Web site maintained by a society of otolaryngologists who focus on rhinology has information for patients on sinusitis and nasal and sinus surgeries.

Asthma and Allergy Foundation of America

1233 20th Street, NW
Suite 402
Washington, DC 20036
1-800-7ASTHMA (1-800-727-8462)
www.aafa.org

Patient information is available on this Web site, as well as a directory of support groups.

Cystic Fibrosis Foundation

6931 Arlington Road
Bethesda, MD 20814
1-800-FIGHT-CF (1-800-344-4823)
www.cff.org

This Web site has a broad variety of information for patients regarding treatment and research on cystic fibrosis.

Foundation for Sarcoidosis Research
122 South Michigan Avenue
Suite 1700
Chicago, IL 60603
312-341-0500
www.stopsarcoidosis.org
Information on sarcoidosis treatment and research is included on this Web site.

Medline Plus: Sinusitis
http://www.nlm.nih.gov/medlineplus/sinusitis.html#cat22
Medline plus is a service of the National Library of Medicine and National Institutes of Health that brings together reliable information for patients. Links to other Web sites on topics in sinusitis are provided.

National Center for Health Statistics
http://www.cdc.gov/nchs/fastats/sinuses.htm
This Web site provides Statistics on chronic sinusitis compiled by the Centers for Disease Control (CDC).

National Institute of Allergy and Infectious Diseases Sinusitis Fact Sheet
NIAID Office of Communications and Public Liaison
6610 Rockledge Drive, MSC 6612
Bethesda, MD 20892-6612
301-496-5717
www.niaid.nih.gov/factsheets/sinusitis.htm
Some basic information on sinusitis is provided at this website.

National Institutes of Health Clinical Trials Registry
www.clinicaltrials.gov
This is a registry of clinical trials conducted in the United States and is maintained by the National Institutes of Health.

Sinus and Allergy Health Partnership

1990 M Street, NW, Suite 680
Washington, DC 20036
202-955-5010
www.sahp.org

This is a joint project of several medical societies with the goal of promoting more effective treatment of allergies and sinusitis. There is information for patients on sinusitis as well as a healthcare provider directory.

U.S. Food and Drug Administration

5600 Fishers Lane
Rockville, MD 20857-0001
1-888-INFO-FDA (1-888-463-6332)
www.fda.gov

This is the Web site for the government agency that oversees drug manufacturing in the United States.

U.S. National Library of Medicine

www.pubmed.gov

This is a Web site that allows a search of articles published, listing the medical journals by subject and author.

Vasculitis Foundation

Wegener's Granulomatosis Association
P.O. Box 28660
Kansas City, MO 64188-8660
1-800-277-9474
www.vasculitisfoundation.org

This is an umbrella organization for a group of 35 related disorders including Wegener's granulomatosis, with information for patients and links to support groups.

Glossary

A

Acupressure: Technique based on restoring the balance of the body's life force by stimulating specific points with pressure.

Acupuncture: A technique based on restoring the balance of the body's life force by stimulating specific points with needles.

Acute sinusitis: Sinus infections that last less than 6 weeks.

Adenoids: Hump of lymphoid tissue in the back of the nose.

Adenoidectomy: Removal of enlarged lymphoid tissue present in the back of the nose.

Allergic fungal sinusitis: Form of sinusitis that is characterized by an allergy to fungus, nasal polyps, and the presence of allergic mucin, a thick peanut butter-like mucus.

Allergist: Physician who specializes in the evaluation and management of allergic disease.

Allergy immunotherapy: A progressive series of injections containing increasing amounts of a substance to which the doctor is attempting to desensitize the patient.

Allergic rhinitis: An inflammation of the lining of the nose triggered by a substance to which sensitivity has been acquired.

Anaphylaxis: Life-threatening systemic allergic reaction that can cause the closure of breathing passageways.

Antibiotics: Class of medications that inhibit or kill bacterial microorganisms

Aqueous nasal sprays: Nasal spray formulations that are water-based.

Aspirin triad: See *Samter's triad.*

Asthma: A disorder in which the lungs become inflamed and constrict in response to triggers such as dust, pollens, pollution, cold temperatures, or exercise.

B

Bacteria: A type of microorganism that can cause infection.

Balloon sinuplasty: A form of sinus surgery in which small balloons are used to dilate sinus openings.

Biofilms: Aggregates of bacteria that have been implicated in the pathogenesis of some forms of sinusitis.

C

Capsaicin: Chemical component of plants present in hot peppers that can be an irritant to skin and mucosa, but may also have topical analgesic properties.

Cavernous sinus thrombosis: Complication of sinusitis that occurs when the sinus infection extends into the blood vessels behind the sphenoid sinus.

Cerebrospinal fluid (CSF) leak: Leakage of the fluid that the brain normally floats within.

Chronic sinusitis: Persistent sinus infection and inflammation lasting 12 weeks or more.

Cilia: Microscopic hairs on the surface of the mucosa lining of the nose and sinuses that beat in a synchronized fashion to help sweep away mucus and debris.

Concha bullosa: Pneumatized turbinate bone that can widen the turbinate and narrow sinus drainage pathways.

Culture: Obtaining a sample of infected material and sending it to the laboratory to identify causative organisms.

Cystic fibrosis (CF): Recessive inherited disorder causing abnormalities in the lungs, sinuses, pancreas, liver, and reproductive tract.

D

Decongestants: Medications that shrink the lining of the nose by constricting blood vessels.

Drug–drug interactions: When one drug affects how another works.

Dura: Thick, tough covering that surrounds and protects the brain.

E

Endoscope: Thin fiberoptic rigid or flexible viewing tube with a lighted lens on one end and eyepiece on the other used to examine surfaces inside the body, such as the inside of the nose, through an orifice such as a nostril.

Endorphins: Naturally occurring chemicals that bind the same areas as narcotics, thereby relieving pain.

Ethmoid sinus: Sinus composed of many small cells located between the eyes.

F

Fascia: Connective tissue that covers, separates, or connects together muscles, organs, and other tissues.

Fluoroscopy: The use of X-ray to produce an image on a monitor in real-time, rather than printing on film.

Frontal sinus: Sinus located in the forehead above the eyes.

Functional endoscopic sinus surgery (FESS): Minimally invasive form of sinus surgery that attempts to restore normal sinus drainage pathways.

Fungus ball: Form of fungal sinusitis also called a *mycetoma*, which is a collection of fungal debris within a sinus.

G

Gastroesophageal reflux disease (GERD): Occurs when gastric acid and enzymes from the stomach back up inside the esophagus.

General anesthesia: Form of anesthesia in which the patient is completely asleep and breathing is assisted by a ventilator.

I

Image-guidance system: computer navigation system for surgery that helps provide the surgeon with additional anatomical information.

Invasive fungal sinusitis: Aggressive form of fungal sinusitis that develops in immunocompromised patients and diabetic patients; it rapidly destroys tissue and can spread to the brain and the eye.

Inverted papilloma: Noncancerous, but aggressively growing tumor of the nose and sinuses.

L

Laryngopharyngeal reflux: Occurs when the acid and enzymes from the stomach leak up the esophagus all the way to the larynx (voice box).

M

Malignant hyperthermia: Life-threatening high body temperature and muscle rigidity in response to certain anesthetic medications; runs in families.

Maxillary sinus: Sinus located in the cheeks on either side of the nose.

Maximal medical therapy: Using the most extensive courses and optimal combinations of medications possible for treatment.

Meningitis: Infection of the tissues that cover and surround the brain.

Microdebriders: Sinus surgery instrument that sucks tissue into it and removes the tissue with a spinning blade.

Middle meatal spacer: Non-absorbable material inserted in the space between the middle turbinate and the side of the nasal cavity to help prevent collapse of the middle turbinate.

Migraine: Severe form of headaches, often one-sided that can be mistaken for a sinus headache; can be associated with light sensitivity, nausea, or postnasal drip.

Mold: Fungus; plants that make spores instead of seeds.

Mucin: Thick, greenish material produced in the sinuses in allergic fungal sinusitis.

Mucocoele: Mucus-filled collection.

Mucociliary clearance: The process by which mucus and materials caught within it are moved from the nose and sinuses by the cilia to the back of the throat.

Mucolytics: Medications that help to thin mucus secretions and make them easier to clear.

Mucus: Fluid secreted from the cells lining the nose and sinuses.

Mucosal membrane: Thin layer of tissue that lines normal nose and sinuses.

Myofascial release: Manual massage technique used to eliminate pain and restore motion.

N

Nasal packing: Sponge-like or ribbon-like material placed in the nose to help stop bleeding.

Nasal polyps: Pink, watery growths that can develop in the nose and sinuses.

Nasal saline irrigation: Flushing the nose with a large volume of salt solution.

Nasal septum: Wall made of bone and cartilage that separates the two sides of the nose.

Navigational scans: Type of CT scan performed using a specific protocol for image-guided surgery.

Nebulizer: A machine that blows the medications into a mist that is deposited on the walls of the nose and sinuses.

Neuralgias: Intense burning or stabbing pain caused by irritation or damage to a nerve.

Neuritis: An inflammation of nerve endings that triggers pain.

Non-allergic rhinitis: Nasal congestion, sneezing, and runny nose triggered by non-allergens such as chemical irritants, hormones, infections, or drugs.

O

Optic nerve: Nerve that transmits signals from the eye to the brain.

Orbit: Eye socket and its contents.

Orbital abscess: Complication of sinusitis in which a collection of infected pus develops within the fat or muscles of the eye socket.

Ostia: Small openings from the sinuses into the nasal cavities.

P

Preseptal cellulitis: Complication of sinusitis that develops when sinus infections extend to the skin and soft tissue surrounding the eye.

Primary ciliary dyskinesia: Genetic disorder causing defective cilia to be unable to beat effectively.

R

Radioallergosorbent test (RAST): Blood test that measures the amount of an antibody that your body makes to fight a particular allergen to determine if you are allergic to it.

Rhinitis medicamentosa: Condition in which overuse of topical decongestant nasal sprays causes the lining of the nose to be nearly persistently congested due to rebound congestion.

Rhinoplasty: Cosmetic surgery to alter the external appearance of the nose.

S

Saddle nose: Depression of the nasal dorsum caused by destruction of the cartilage of the nasal septum.

Samter's triad: Also called the *aspirin triad*; comprised of aspirin allergy, asthma, and nasal polyps.

Sarcoidosis: A rare disease that causes beads of inflamed tissue to form in the body.

Septoplasty: Surgery to correct the crooked areas of the nasal septum.

Sinuses: Hollow air-filled cavities located in the head.

Sinusitis: Disease characterized by inflammation of the mucosa lining the sinuses.

Sphenoid sinus: Sinus located deep inside the head, under the brain and behind the eyes.

Squamous cell carcinoma: Form of cancer that arises from the cells on the skin or lining the surfaces of the gastrointestinal and respiratory tracts.

Steroids: A class of medications with strong anti-inflammatory properties.

Subperiosteal abscess: Complication of sinusitis in which infection of the skin around the eye spreads to the bone within the eye socket.

T

Topical antibiotics: Form of antibiotics delivered directly to the tissues they are treating in spray, irrigation, or nebulized forms.

Turbinates: Scrolls of bone covered with mucosa that extend from the nasal walls inside the nose that humidify and warm the air as it passes through the nasal passageway.

Turbinate reduction: Surgery to reduce the size of the inferior turbinates.

W

Wegener's granulomatosis: A rare disease that causes clumps of inflamed tissue to form throughout the body.

V

Vasomotor rhinitis: Abnormal response to stimuli such as heat, cold, or spicy foods that results in nasal congestion and rhinorrhea.

X

Xylitol: Type of sugar alcohol that has antibacterial properties.

Italic page numbers refer to illustrations.